The Fear Factor: How Stigma Hinders the Fight Against HIV in MSM

Fedor

CONTENTS

PART 3 RESULTS

PART 4 DISCUSSIONS AND CONCLUSION

PART 1. INTRODUCTION

1.1 Statement of the Problem

The Human Immunodeficiency Virus (HIV) represents one of the world's most serious public health challenges. In 2020, approximately 38 million people were living with HIV around the world. Of these, 7.8 million did not yet know their status. In 2019, an estimated 1,7 million individuals worldwide acquired HIV, marking a 40% decline compared to the peak in 1998. As of the end of 2020, 26 million people were accessing antiretroviral therapy (ART), meaning that more than 12 million are still waiting (1).

To better monitor global progress, the term "continuum of HIV services" has been adopted by the World Health Organization (WHO) and used internationally. It refers to the sequence of steps a person with HIV takes from diagnosis through receiving treatment until his or her viral load is suppressed to undetectable levels. Each step in the continuum is marked by an assessment of the number of people who have reached that stage. The stages are: being diagnosed with HIV; being linked to medical care; starting ART; adhering to the treatment regimen; and, finally, having HIV suppressed to undetectable levels in the blood. The joint United Nations Program on HIV/AIDS (UNAIDS)'s 90-90-90 goals set as targets that by 2020, 90% of all people with HIV will know their HIV status, 90% of all people who know their status will be on ART, and 90% of all people receiving ART will have viral suppression. As presented in figure 1, tracking progress toward those goals, UNAIDS reports that in 2020, of all people with HIV worldwide: 81% knew their HIV status, 67% were accessing ART and 59% were virally suppressed (1).

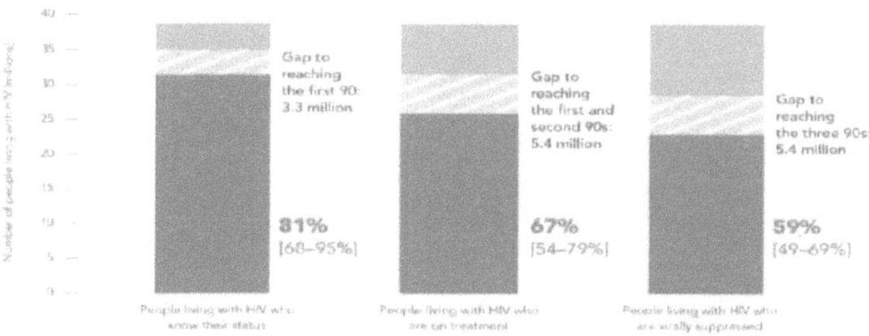

Figure 1. 2020 global HIV testing and treatment cascade (UNAIDS, 2020).

Despite advances in scientific understanding of HIV and its prevention and treatment as well as years of significant effort by the global health community and leading government and civil society organizations, too many people with HIV or at risk for HIV still do not have access to prevention, care, and treatment, and there is still no cure. Stigma and discrimination, together with other social inequalities and exclusion, are proving to be key barriers since the beginning of the epidemic (2). Stigma against people living with HIV (PLHIV), especially sexual minorities, reinforces marginalization and makes access to care difficult and results in loss to follow-up (LTFU) (3). According to Canadian sociologist Ervin Goffman (1963), one of the earliest scholars to theorize stigma, it is any personal attribute, real or perceived, that conveys a negative social identity, thus devaluing the person's social position (4). Specific to HIV, the UNAIDS describes stigma as "a process of devaluation of people either living with, or associated with, HIV and acquired immunodeficiency syndrome (AIDS)" (5). This condition is considered as one of the major barriers to effective responses to the HIV epidemic and despite public education programs and equal rights legislation, stigmatization continues to be widespread and affect many aspects of life (6, 7).

Men who have sex with men (MSM) are among the community populations throughout the world that have been one of the constituencies most affected by HIV, and continue to be one of the population groups most vulnerable to infection and death related to HIV. Due to biological, behavioral and social factors, MSM are 27 times more at risk for HIV and the 2020 data, presented in figure 2, showed that they accounted for 23% of new infections (8–10).

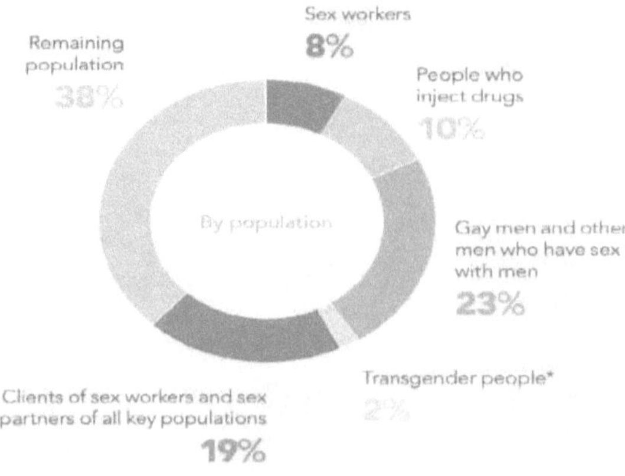

Figure 2. Distribution of new HIV infections by population group (UNAIDS, 2020).

MSM living with HIV are subjected to a plethora of unpleasant treatment that includes discrimination, social ostracism and violence (11). Globally, 69 countries have laws that criminalize same-sex sexual relations. As a result, the social, emotional and relational aspects of their lives are sometimes extremely affected, leading to marginalization (3). In addition to this, stigmatization linked to homosexuality and fear of being HIV-positive present barriers to making use of the available voluntary HIV testing and counseling services (12). Experienced stigma is the actual experience or occurrence of discrimination, such as denial of health care services or the criminalization of same-sex practices. These forms of stigma play a significant role in the lives of MSM and within the context of the HIV epidemic (13). A review of the literature suggests that MSM are inadequately studied in many countries, and that despite well-characterized risks for HIV acquisition and transmission, MSM continue to be under-represented in national HIV surveillance systems, in targeted prevention programs, and in care (14). The global response to the pandemic has progressed over the decades both in scale and in efforts to reach diverse and vulnerable groups, stigma and discrimination still follow affected MSM in many settings (13).

PLHIV are often victims of adverse behavior in relation to their status. A despised label is therefore attributed, making them, sometimes, unconsciously victims. These same attitudes are also found in the face of a sexual orientation different from what society or political and religious norms describe as normal. Hence the effect of "double victim" perceived by MSM infected with HIV (15). These reactions have been described as "stigmatization". According to Erving Goffman, stigma is defined as "any characteristic of the individual which, if known, discredits him in the eyes of others or makes him appear to be a person of lesser status" (4). Several interpretations and definitions of HIV-related stigma have been developed (6,16–18).

The fear of MSM living with HIV to health care structures hinders the success of health and social interventions. This has been demonstrated in several countries as the epidemic continues to increase among sexual minorities. Homophobia is the product of deeply rooted views of specific roles, religion, and identity. (13,19,20). In many developing societies, arguments for recognizing sexual diversity and gender are considered as imposing Western models of individualism (21).

Before reaching Haiti, a focus on the Caribbean region showed the global HIV prevalence was 1.1% and 330.000 people were living with HIV in 2019. Haiti alone accounted for nearly half of them. As shown in figure 3, out of the 13.000 new infections reported that year, MSM represented nearly a quarter. Besides, HIV prevalence among MSM was over 15% in Trinidad and Tobago, Bahamas and Haiti. Thus, MSM are the group most affected by HIV in the region (1, 5). Several factors are behind this high burden. Although sex between men is rather frequent in the region, male homosexual behavior does not usually imply homosexual or bisexual self-identities (6, 7). Homosexuality is still a source of stigma, discrimination and human rights violations in many islands (8). Many MSM fear public exposure, social rejection and are likely to access healthcare or social services late in their disease course if at all (24,25).

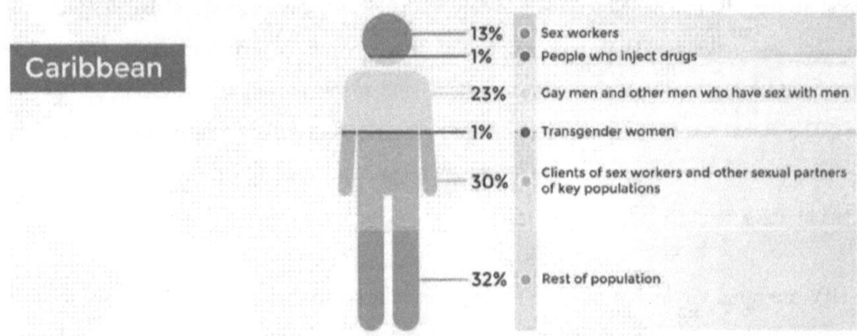

Figure 3. Distribution of new HIV infections by population groups in the Caribbean (AVERT, UNAIDS, 2020).

HIV first emerged in Haiti in the late 1970s. But, by 1982, the Centers for Disease Control (CDC) named four groups as "risk factors" for HIV infection: homosexuals, heroin addicts, hemophiliacs and Haitians. The stigma conferred by the new disease on all these groups - who were designated in the popular press as "the 4H Club" - was immediate and severe (26).

In 2019, for a prevalence of 2.2%, about 160.000 people were living with HIV in Haiti. Although the exact number of MSM is not estimated due to disclosure issues, HIV prevalence was 18.2% in 2017 according to the UNAIDS. Tracking progress toward the 90-90-90 goals, in 2019 of the 160,000 PLHIV: 72% knew their HIV status, 71% were accessing ART and 56% were virally suppressed (1).

The poorest country in the Western hemisphere, Haiti has the highest number of people living with HIV in the Caribbean, the second most affected region in the world outside of Africa in terms of prevalence (26). Despite many public health interventions in the region and nationwide, PLHIV in Haiti are vulnerable to stigmatization, particularly sexual minorities. The latter suffer considerable ostracism, which prevents access to care. Sometimes extreme marginalization also affects the social, emotional and relational aspects of their life. New prevention and treatment opportunities are likely to be unavailable for many MSM, who are stigmatized, persecuted and ignored by the new law prohibiting same-sex marriage and the promotion of homosexuality (6-8, 26).

Yet, on August 2017, the Haitian Senate passed a law prohibiting marriage between same-sex couples. While this measure is not new – as the national civil code recognizes only the unions between a man and a woman – the vote reflects a growing intolerance towards the MSM community, because it aims to prohibit any display of homosexuality in the public space. In addition, there is no anti-hate crime law that specifically addresses the discrimination and harassment experienced by MSM because of their sexual orientation or gender identity. Homosexuality is considered taboo by Haitians who are largely influenced by Christianity. Weaknesses in government and legal structures – including the penal system – also contribute to stigmatize and discriminate against people living with HIV. A proposal in December 2011 of a law to the Haitian Parliament to better protect people living with HIV against stigma and discrimination hasn't been considered so far (24, 25, 27).

Special statement of the problem in regards to the current COVID-19 pandemic

As the past cannot be rewritten, imagining a better future with respect to the actual coronavirus pandemic should allow the global health community to frame a world with less stigma towards the end of HIV. Unfortunately, COVID-19 exposed, once again, the deep roots of inequalities: *"Sexual minorities have previously been blamed for several disasters, both man-made and natural. At the start of the HIV epidemic, in many countries gay men were frequently stigmatized and abused because they were believed to be responsible for transmitting HIV. Also, in the current context of the COVID-19 pandemic, several reports mentioned by the UNAIDS, suggest that LGBTQ + people are held responsible for this scourge and that they are suffering an increase in discriminatory acts. In addition, due to movement restrictions and social distancing measures in force, sexual minorities are also confined in sometimes hostile family and community environments. This can increase their exposure to violence and abuse without being able to proceed with legal actions due to fear of repercussions, thus exacerbating their pre-existing vulnerabilities to HIV."* Willy Dunbar & Yves Coppieters; Le Covid-19 suscite une nouvelle stigmatisation des personnes LGBT+. *The Conversation* (2021).

1.2 Stigma: Definition and Conceptualization

As a process of devaluation that excludes, rejects, blames or devalues individuals in the eyes of others, the definition of "stigma" is variable in the literature (28,29).

Erving Goffman provided a seminal theorization of health-related stigma in the 1960s through his work in psychiatric hospitals and among criminals and homosexuals (30). He defined stigma as "an attribute that is deeply discrediting," and that reduces the bearer "from a whole and usual person to a tainted, discounted one" (30). Based on his work, the society stigmatizes on the basis of what is constituted as "difference" or "deviance," and results in a "spoiled identity" (17,30). The social label of deviance compels stigmatized individuals to view themselves and others, to view the stigmatized as discredited or undesirable (6). Daily routines establish the usual and the expected, certain appearances help us anticipate what Goffman called "social identity." (31).

Goffman distinguished three types of stigma: physical deformity, character blemishes and prejudice. The second one may occur in individuals with HIV. For example, individuals living with HIV face considerable stigma because many believe that the infected person could have controlled the behaviors that resulted in the infection (4). In addition to this, some groups, identities, and behaviors are consistently stigmatized across much of the world. Examples include stigma based on: sexual practices and identities of gay men and other MSM (32-34). In many cases, for MSM, HIV poses a double burden—on the one hand, there are a very limited number of programs specifically designed to reach them, and on the other hand, they are often faced with discrimination, stigma and in some cases even criminal prosecution by the societies they live in (1).

Psychologists and sociologists have built on Goffman's theory to address the concepts of felt stigma and enacted stigma. Felt stigma is an internalized perception of being devalued or "not as good as" by an individual. Enacted stigma on the other hand refers to behaviors and perceptions by others toward the individual who is perceived as different (32,33). Stigma is, thus, enacted and perceived through social processes, violence, aggression and family rejection (35).

Besides Goffman's works, Earnshaw and Chaudoir proposed a HIV stigma Framework. This framework suggests that the social phenomenon of HIV stigma impacts individual PLWH via a series of HIV stigma mechanisms, which are distinct psychological responses to the knowledge that they possess a socially devalued characteristic. Based on Earnshaw and Chaudoir works, "People who are living with HIV know that their status is an extremely socially devalued aspect of the self, and this knowledge is experienced through at least three important stigma forms: enacted stigma, anticipated stigma, and internalized stigma. Enacted stigma refers to the degree to which people believe they have actually experienced prejudice and discrimination from others in their community. Anticipated stigma refers to the degree to which people expect that they will experience prejudice and discrimination from others in the future. Internalized stigma refers to the degree to which people endorse the negative beliefs and feelings associated with HIV about themselves" (36,37).

This dynamic concept is approached from different theoretical views that led to different conceptualizations. Link defined stigma as a social process that exists when elements of labelling, stereotyping, separation, status loss, and discrimination occur in a power situation that allows them (16). Weiss and Ramakrishna went further by describing it as a related personal experience characterized by exclusion, rejection, blame or devaluation that results from experience or reasonable anticipation of an adverse social judgement about a person or group. In health-related stigma, this judgment is based on an enduring feature of identity conferred by a health problem or health related condition (38).

A link from socio-anthropological theory to public health in understanding stigma and discrimination bring us to the complex systems of beliefs about HIV and other diseases that are often grounded in social inequalities (39). Theoretical frameworks to understanding HIV stigma have been developed ethnographically in many countries including Haiti (40). Although the first references to the association between stigma and health in the social science literature date back to the 1880s, Goffman, beginning with his work in psychiatric hospitals in the late 1950s, institutionalized the benchmark social theory of the association between stigma and disease. Others have used a similar approach to understanding stigma associated with diseases such as hookworm, tuberculosis, cancer, polio, and sexually transmitted infections and the association of these diseases with racist ideology in the United States (41).

The field of social psychology and anthropology have noted the cognitive considerations that lead to labeling and stereotyping. However, most research in these fields focuses more on attitudes, perceptions and views from individuals rather than a complex social ground as they referred to misunderstandings and misinformation when it comes to behavioral changes. While some anthropologists have neglected the social inequalities behind the structural violence by prioritizing cognitivist interpretations, others have taken precautions to make sure that lived experience informed their interpretations (42). These findings reinforced our works by proving that the fundamental causes of stigma need to be addressed by targeting multiple mechanisms to bring change.

Although stigma is a multidisciplinary concept, one of the major issues is the existence of valid and reliable scales that consider different aspects and layers like enacted, anticipated and internalized in PLHIW and MSM. Some scales have been developed, tested and validated. Others have been adapted regarding the population groups and socio-cultural contexts. Some researchers used multiple HSS or parts of different scales. In terms of reliability of the instrument, Cronbach's alpha is widely used. Alpha was developed by Lee Cronbach in 195 to provide a measure of the internal consistency of a test or scale and it is expressed as a number between 0 and 1. Other instruments include items from the Attitudes Toward Lesbians and Gay Men (ATLG) which was originally developed in 1984 and revised several times, the Reactions to Homosexuality Scale and the Modern Homonegativity Scale (MHS) (43).

We present a summary of the most used scales:

- Berger et al.'s 40-item HIV Stigma Scale is the most commonly used and is one of only a few scales that cover the different mechanisms. Psychometric analysis was performed on 318 questionnaires returned by people with HIV (19% women, 21% African American, 8% Hispanic). Four factors emerged from exploratory factor analysis: personalized stigma, disclosure concerns, negative self-image, and concern with public attitudes toward people with HIV. Cronbach's alphas were provided for total scale score (0.94) as well as disclosure concerns (0.79), personalized stigma (0.93), negative self-image (0.84) and public attitudes (0.91) subscales (44). Other scales include:

- Swendeman et al. modified a pre-existing scale with questions characterized by factors of avoidance, social rejections, abuse and shame. It resulted in 11 enacted stigma item and 7 perceived stigma items (45).
- The seven perceived items utilized by Radcliffe et al. to assess stigma among young MSM in the United States. The response format was altered to yes/no, but items were not otherwise altered, and no factor analyses or Cronbach's alphas were reported (46).
- In Africa, Mavhu et al. used a mixed methods approach to assess HIV stigma using a quantitative measure that was developed from questionnaires previously validated as well as newly developed and pretested questions. Factor analysis and Cronbach's alpha were not mentioned for this measure of stigma (47).
- In China, Zhao et al. developed new questions to assess attitudes toward PLHIV. The 10 questions were developed from a literature review on HIV stigma and had a Cronbach's alpha of 0.87 (48).
- Ha et al. developed and assessed a homosexuality-related stigma scale among MSM in Vietnam by conducting a cross-sectional study using respondent-driven sampling. Factor analysis was performed, and interitem correlation matrices were constructed to identify the latent factor structures, examine the goodness of fit, and assess convergent and discriminant validity of the determined scales (49).
- Klein et al developed the PrEP stigma scale to try to understand why MSM are not adopting PrEP in greater numbers, by created a 22-item PrEP Stigma Scale (50).

1.3 Intersection of HIV Stigma and Homonegativity

Since the beginning of the HIV epidemic, stigma and discrimination have been barriers to proper responses and have greatly exacerbated the negative impact of the epidemic. Indeed, the stigma and discrimination associated with HIV continues to manifest in all countries and in all regions of the world and is a major obstacle to preventing new infections, mitigating the impact and providing adequate care, support and treatment (51–53).

Stigma associated with HIV has cut short the debate about both causes and responses. Visibility and openness about the Acquired Immunodeficiency Syndrome (AIDS) problem are prerequisites for effective mobilization of government, community and individual resources that can change the epidemic. Concealing the problem may lead to denying its existence and refusing to recognize that action must be taken quickly. This can lead to PLHIV being wrongly considered as a kind of problem rather than a solution to contain and manage the epidemic. The stigma associated with HIV is caused by all sorts of factors, including a misunderstanding of the disease, myths about HIV transmission, inadequate access to treatment, the irresponsible way in which the media talks about the epidemic, the fact that AIDS is incurable, as well as prejudices and fears related to a number of socially sensitive issues such as sexuality, illness and death, and drug use (54,55).

From the insidious, silent start towards the end of the 70s, the beginning of the 80s of this pandemic that was going to become the evil of the century, its manifestations, its morbidity and its mortality strongly linked to the difficulties of discovering its causal agent, its modes of transmission and its origin have permanently built the foundations of this stigma and discrimination that would cause so much harm to those infected and / or affected and especially to the pursuit of a global response to the dimensions of this thorny problem (37,53). Thus, all over the world, particularly in Haiti, at very different levels, we have observed and unfortunately still observe well-documented cases of PLHIV who are ostracized and discriminated against and who see each other denying access to services because of their HIV status, in the workplace, in the areas of education and health care, and even in communities surrounding PLHIV (56,57). They also reduce prevention efforts because people are afraid to discover that they are infected or not, in order to seek treatment, for fear of the reactions of others. They push those who are at risk of infection and some of those who are affected to continue to practice unprotected sexuality because they think that by changing their behavior they will raise doubts about their HIV status (58).

Stigma is considered as social devaluation of a person based on an attribute, and discrimination as behavior resulting from harm. Sexual stigma, commonly defined as a shared belief system that denigrates and discredits homosexuality versus heterosexuality, affects the lives of homosexuals and other MSM (20). Populations at risk for HIV infection experience stigma. This is especially true for MSM, who are often blamed for the epidemic itself because many were infected in the beginning and traditional attitudes toward homosexuality and corresponding views of promiscuity, moral degeneracy, and being "diseased" (59). HIV related stigma has implications for the health of yet uninfected MSM at risk for HIV infection and for incidence and prevalence of the disease itself. For example, HIV related stigma makes it difficult for MSM to initiate safer sex practices because doing so implies that your partner is "unclean." Conversely, requesting the use of a condom can also as easily imply that the one making the request is "unclean." (60).

Highly stigmatized by both religious and social norms, homosexual practices are driven underground. Some men are involved with both male and female sexual partners. And sometimes they appear to adopt a socially acceptable heterosexual lifestyle. Marrying women and fathering children are, for some, a strategy to avoid negative consequences of public disclosure of homosexuality and can be used to help dispel doubts about masculinity. By having female sexual partners, MSM fulfil the traditional gender roles and respect the heteronormative and hegemonic model of masculinity (61). In this way, structural factors are interconnected and converge to increased individual risk practices, thus increasing both social and other individual drivers of HIV vulnerability. Additionally, HIV related stigma and discrimination may deter individuals from seeking information and assistance for risk reduction practices and supplies (62).

1.4 HIV Epidemic in Haiti

As presented in the statement of problem, Haiti has the largest number of people living with HIV in the Caribbean, the most affected region in the world outside of Africa in terms of prevalence (63). Despite ongoing political, socio-economic and natural disasters, Haiti remains committed to the fight against the HIV epidemic. The government's prevention and treatment strategies in collaboration with nongovernmental organizations have contributed to reducing the national prevalence of HIV, from 6.2% in 1993 to 2.2 % since 2016 (64). The strength and HIV program resistance in Haiti are also highlighted by the response to the January 2010 earthquake, which left more than 15% of the population homeless, and destroyed government offices, health facilities and homes. But, in just a few months after, the number of patients on ARV across the country was over 90% of the pre-quake level. A recent national study suggests that HIV prevalence has not increased over the four years after the earthquake, remaining at 2.2% (64,65). Shortly after the disaster, Haiti experienced a major cholera epidemic, which also had no negative impact on the HIV care system by impacting regular services (66,67).

Unfavorable environments identified at the health facility and community level hinder the continuum of care. This stigma sometimes translates into humiliation, blackmail and violence. As a result, the smooth running of the program is hampered. The Haitian government and the private sector are not yet active in defending the rights of MSM and promoting a safer legal and social environment to reduce discrimination and stigmatization. Thus, the survey conducted by the UNAIDS revealed that HIV prevalence among MSM is 18.2% (68,69-74).

According to the International Refugee Right Initiative, there is no law against homosexuality in the Haitian Penal Code. As a minimum, Haitian MSM are protected under the 1987 Constitution: art. 35-2, which prohibits discrimination in the workplace on the basis of "sex, opinions and marital status". Haiti does not recognize same-sex marriage, civil union or common-law marriage. However, the current situation did not stop the Haitian Senate to pass the 2017 law banning same-sex marriage while the draft law for protection of PLHIV submitted to Parliament on 1 December 2011 has not been even considered (68,70,71).

There is no anti-hate crime law that specifically addresses the discrimination and harassment that MSM have to endure because of their sexual orientation or gender identity. Homosexuality is considered taboo by Haitians largely influenced by the Christian religion. On the juridical level, it should be pointed out that the governance structures of the judicial system are weak. Stigma and discrimination against people living with HIV are present.

While the national response to the HIV epidemic has made headway, infected and affected people continue to be stigmatized and discriminated both in the community and in healthcare settings (9). Infected and high-risk individuals are often perceived as socially despised behaviors, such as homosexual practices (72,73).

Efforts have been undertaken, at all levels of the health system, to ensure proper inclusion of MSM in the HIV response in Haiti by accelerating, delivering and optimizing services that reduce HIV transmission among MSM and prolong life of those who are HIV-positive. Interventions are tailored to the continuum of HIV care focused on prevention, care and treatment (Prevention – Testing - Enrollment in Care – ART initiation - Adherence - Viral Suppression). The approach taken to promote the delivery of prevention services is community-based including peer education, community mobilization and mass awareness of HIV prevention, gender-based violence, stigma and discrimination (74).

Among the leading institutions in the field of HIV prevention and treatment for MSM is the Haitian Group for Kaposi Sarcoma and Opportunistic Infections Study (GHESKIO) in Port-au-Prince. One of the largest institutions dedicated to the fight against HIV / AIDS, GHESKIO has been providing care, research and training in Haiti since 1982. Management of MSM living with HIV is carried out according to the standard model developed by the continuum HIV services including prevention, counselling, testing, enrollment on ART and ongoing follow-up (75).

However, according to the observations and analyzes of the coordination team of care at the national level, the objectives set for counseling, screening, enrollment on ART are never achieved, particularly because of the difficulties related to lack of interventions regarding the social and structural specificities of MSM (56,65). In addition, evaluations have found that health care providers sometimes carry stigma and lack specific skills to meet the needs of this target group (76).

Therefore, operational research, pilot tests of new interventions and further analysis are needed in order to identify the strengths and weaknesses of the health system, the contextual factors in order to propose hypotheses of change for capacity building, regulations and policing measures aiming at reducing inequalities and strengthening social safety through engagement, adherence and retention.

1.5 The Haitian Health System: Focus on HIV Care

In order to achieve its objectives, the Haitian health system has a set of means to make available its range of health services. Care is provided by four types of institutions depending on the type of management. These are establishments in the sectors:

• Public (under the State)

• Private for-profit

• Private non-profit

• Mixed (where the public and private sectors co-manage)

There are institutions that support the health system. These are the paramedical institutions and training institutions (77).

Haiti's Health Policy, developed in 1996, recognizes the fundamental right of every person to receive preventive and curative health care regardless of discrimination. In addition, the holistic approach to health in the provision of services has been advocated so that the individual is considered in his existential life and has at his disposal a complete range of services to enable him to maintain his health. So, health policy is based on principles of equity, social justice and solidarity even though access to care is not free (78-80).

The Haitian health system is represented by the national health authorities, the central authorities, the departmental levels, the communal offices and the care facilities, all of which are distributed within the Ministry of Public Health and Population. Entities specifically responsible for the delivery of services are health institutions (public, private or mixed). This offer of formal care is extended to only 47% of the population. This reduced access is partially offset by the use of traditional medicine as a first resort to diseases including HIV. The private health sector is very important, especially the for-profit one. Funding sources for medical care come from international aid at 64%, households at 29% and government budget participation only 7 (78-80).

HIV funders in Haiti are the Government of Haiti, the US President's Emergency Plan for AIDS Relief (PEPFAR), the United States Agency for International Development (USAID) and the multilateral sector through the United Nations (UN). Many challenges exist at the systems level, particularly from the point of view of governance, coordination and human resource management (77).

As the 2020 data showed, MSM are 27 times more at risk for HIV than the general population. Besides, they accounted for 23% of new infections. The high probability of HIV transmission from condom-free receptive sex converges with socio-cultural factors and multiple partners, making care even more complex (1, 81-83). The continuum of services takes the form of preventive educational activities, distribution of condoms and lubricants, screening and integrated treatment for HIV and other sexually transmitted infections (STIs). Sites of care are also effective places to treat victims of gender-based violence and accidental exposure to blood. This model includes the following steps: identification, linkage, screening, diagnosis, enrollment, ART initiation, adherence and viral suppression (64).

Medically, sustained attention is given to the new principles of the WHO: "test and treatment". Mathematical models have shown that such a strategy could reduce HIV transmission especially in high prevalence communities, assuming high management and adherence to ARV. Thus, to optimize the care for MSM, Haiti started in 2016 the Linkages Across the Continuum of HIV Services for MSM Affected by HIV (LINKAGES) Project (76).

1.6 Linkages Across the Continuum of HIV Services for MSM Affected by HIV (LINKAGES) Project

The Linkages Across the Continuum of HIV Services for Key populations for HIV (KP) including MSM Affected by HIV (LINKAGES) Project aims to accelerate the ability of governments, MSM organizations and private sector providers to collaboratively plan, deliver and optimize services that reduce HIV transmission among MSM and their sexual partners and extend life for those who are HIV-positive. This project is led by The Family Health International (FHI 360) with GHESKIO as one of the key partners. Key populations— which include sex workers, people who inject drugs, prisoners, transgender people, and gay men and other men who have sex with men—constitute small proportions of the general population, but they are at elevated risk of acquiring HIV infection, in part due to discrimination and social exclusion.

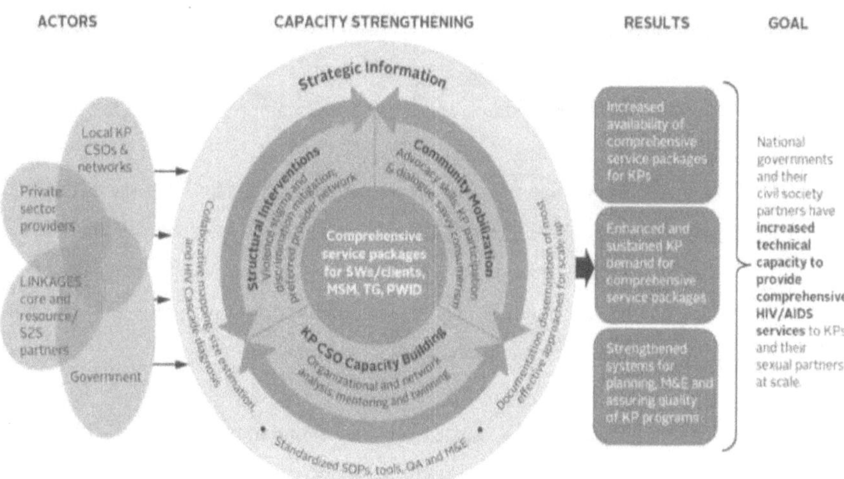

Figure 4. Strategic and technical approach of the LINKAGES (Francis and Mills, 2015)

ART Antiretroviral Therapy - CSO Civil Society Organization - KP Key Population - M&E Monitoring and Evaluation - MSM Men Who Have Sex with Men - PWID People Who Inject Drugs - QA Quality Assurance - SOP Standard Operating Procedure - SW Sex Worker - TG Transgender Individuals

Strategic and technical approach

As described in their framework, FHI 360 and its partners understand that reducing HIV incidence among MSM is complex, risk behaviors are overlapping, and socio-cultural and legal barriers are formidable. For LINKAGES, the team leverages its global technical leadership in MSM programming and record of success in assisting the country to rapidly and sustainably take evidence-based and cost-efficient MSM services to scale. The overarching aim – in line with USAID's goal – is to accelerate the ability of the government, MSM organizations and private sector providers to collaboratively plan, deliver and optimize services that reduce HIV transmission among MSM and their sexual partners and to extend life for those who are HIV-positive.

In addition to its overarching approach, the key elements of the strategic and technical approach are:

- Identifying target populations and locales and comprehensively assessing risk and service access.
- Diagnosing "leaks" and revealing access barriers within the HIV services cascade.
- Scaling up "what works" while innovating to ensure the most strategic use of resources and access to newly emerging technologies.
- Pulling down structural barriers and transforming MSM organizations.
- Ensuring MSM interventions are sustainable over the long term (84).

As presented in Figure 2, the HIV cascade consists of the following stages: 1. Identifying; 2. Reaching; 3. Testing; 4. Diagnosing; 5. Enrolling in care; 6. Initiating ART; 7. Sustaining on ART; 8. Suppressing viral loads. The entire cascade is buttressed by critical environmental, structural, and legal interventions that are designed to help MSM enter and flow through the continuum without fear of stigma, discrimination, arrest, or other adverse consequences (85).

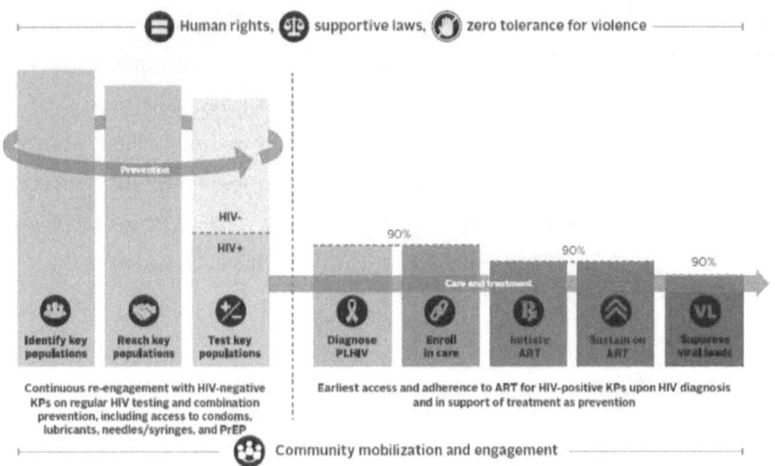

Figure 6. The Continuum of Prevention, Care and Treatment (Francis and Mills, 2015)

The first three bars in the figure represent HIV identification, access and testing in communities at key population levels including MSM and include those who are HIV negative and seronegative. For HIV-negative people, this part of the cascade encompasses primary prevention and underscores the need for continued recommitment to promote prevention approaches that combine rights-based counseling, condom use, regular HIV testing, and infections. sexually transmitted diseases, risk reduction interventions and pre-exposure prophylaxis (PrEP), as appropriate. The remaining bars represent the care and treatment part of the HIV cascade for those who test positive. After a facilitated reference, for example using peer browsers, MSM living with HIV enroll in appropriate care. A dedicated case manager or care team supports PLHIV to access and initiate antiretroviral therapy, providing adherence support to improve health outcomes and, ultimately, reduce viral load (85).

Based on the works of Francis and Mills, MSM face multiple challenges accessing HIV care and adhering to HIV treatment recommendations, including stigma, discrimination, overt violence, a lack of community and social supports and other human rights abuses. Linkages between interventions for MSM are frequently inadequate at every stage of the HIV continuum of prevention, care, and treatment.

These weak linkages among programs can be thought of as a leaky pipe along the continuum of HIV services (Figure 7 below). Outreach programs often refer MSM members to HIV testing and counseling, yet a large segment of those reached never actually go for an HIV test. If they do obtain an HIV test, those who are HIV- negative may only test once or infrequently, despite ongoing risk. Those diagnosed HIV- positive may leave the testing site without a referral to care and treatment. Loss-to- follow-up for MSM is very common across the continuum, contributing to a significant and preventable burden of HIV morbidity and mortality

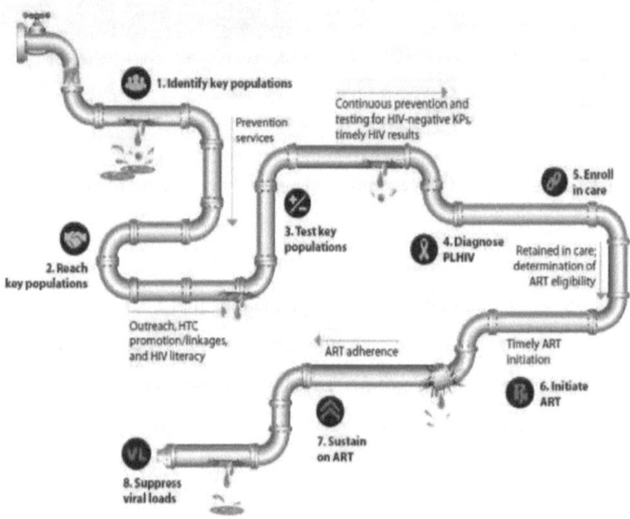

Figure 7. The leaky pipe along the continuum of HIV services (Francis and Mills, 2015)

1.7 The MSM Community in Haiti

A national survey conducted by Population Services International in Haiti (PSI-Haiti) at 12 centers between October and December 2011 identified 54,700 MSM, 82.5% of whom were single, 45.5% considered themselves homosexual and 47.7% as bisexual. The average number of sexual partners per year was estimated at 7. Only 36% could demonstrate adequate use of condoms while 18% had a history of STI that further increases the risk of HIV infection (86). Data from the national program reported in 2019 that the number of identified MSM is 30,900 (1). The inconsistency of those data shows another gap which is the lack of national and subnational-level size estimates for MSM, which are critical to inform national strategy around resource allocation, intervention planning and program evaluation.

Some religious communities, in particular, continue to be homophobic and have a negative impact on education and testing activities, which is a major challenge. MSM refuse to participate because of the insults that are sometimes inflicted on them even by health care providers. In addition, among MSM, several sub-groups are identified: assumed and known homosexuals, hidden homosexuals and bisexuals. Even between these subgroups there is a lot of discrimination and stigmatization. Not only do socio-economic vulnerability and structural barriers increase HIV risk, they also affect care retention and quality of life for MSM living with HIV. Recent findings from the region suggest that inability to pay for care, lack of food and shelter, and depression due to lack of employment opportunities conspire to interrupt HIV care and adversely affect their health (87).

1.8 The Social Accountability of Medical Education

A key concept of the book is the social accountability of medical education regarding the problem of stigma through the healthcare system. Therefore, it is essential to describe it.

The concept of social accountability of medical education is defined as the obligation to improve training in order to meet the needs and challenges of health for citizens and society in general, in accordance with the values of quality, equity, relevance and efficiency. This principle recalls that medical education is geared to the needs and expectations of society first and foremost (88). In light of this reflection and because of the stigmatization perceived by MSM in the healthcare settings, an assessment is needed in order to analyze the implication of the values defended above. Such a reflection should therefore lead us to a focus of medical education on the individual, thereby reducing stigma, marginalization and social inequalities in health. Understanding and testing this social accountability at the professional level and then passing it on to society contributes to achieve the level of understanding and tolerance required to strengthen the continuum of care (89).

"Be socially accountable is to be relevant and efficient in regards to society and the actions that are intended to be carried out in its favor. In the area of health, social accountability is the commitment to respond as effectively as possible to the priority health needs of citizens and society, in particular by establishing the values of quality, equity, relevance and efficiency as founding principles of active participation in the evolution of the health system "(90).

These founding principles refer to an adaptation of basic and continuing medical education according to the real needs and context of society (91). Training future health professionals in adapting their practice according to care seekers and without discrimination is a step to consider in the fight against the stigmatization of MSM. As a result, these better trained professionals will be able to act as agents of change in society not only in terms of service delivery but also in community education and awareness.

1.9 Theoretical framework illustrating how HIV and sexual stigma lead to poor continuum outcomes.

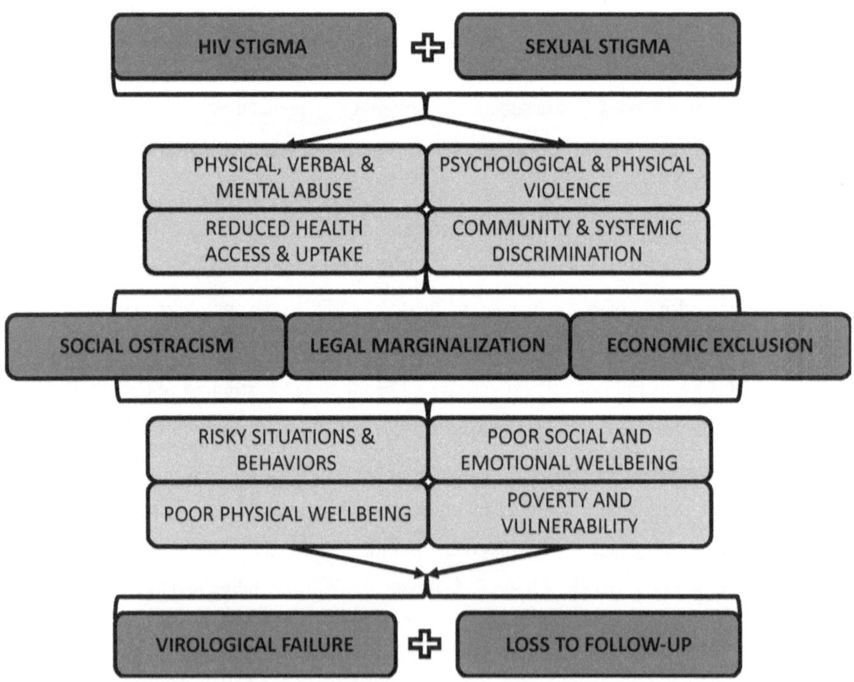

Much of the conceptual frameworks and scientific literature considered stigma as a complex issue when it comes to HIV (92). This complexity is shown by its diversity in different cultural settings as the primary reasons for the failure of implemented interventions and has led to difficulties and disagreement about formal definitions and measurement tools (93). This theoretical framework highlights the impact of stigma on the continuum of HIV services in Haiti through a succession of steps interacting at three different levels.

While irrational, negative attitudes, behaviors, and judgments towards PLHIV have negative impact, they are reinforced when individuals are also subjected to explicit and subtle discrimination and marginalization due to sexual orientation (94). In Haiti, exacerbated by the consequences, the "double victim" effect leads to:

- physical,
- verbal and mental abuse,
- psychological and physical violence,
- community and systemic discrimination, and
- reduced health access and service uptake.

These factors lead to severe social consequences related to human rights, health care services, freedom, self-identity and social interactions. Hence, the effect of social ostracism, legal marginalization and economic exclusion.

Culture and policies impact to the society constitute the footprint of non-tolerance and discrimination that are embedded in the dynamism of Haitian context. MSM are caught in a current situation of social ostracism and violence sometimes generated by leaders, community members and health care providers. Rejection, refusal of help and attack can also come from stigmatized relatives. These reactions influence their behavior in society as well as their education and awareness level to contribute to:

- risky behaviors,
- poor social, emotional and physical wellbeing
- poverty and vulnerability.

The proximal impacts from these reactions are virologic failure and loss to follow-up leading to poor outcomes along the continuum. Considering the context of Haiti, sexuality has long been and is still a taboo subject, even though it has undergone sweeping changes during recent years. On top of that, the emergence of HIV/AIDS, during the past 40 years, has overwhelmed the country. Assessment of the stigma mitigation within a the MSM community suggests the allocation of projects and the use of reliable mechanisms within the communities. A new generation of analysts, an exceptional network of policymakers, thinkers, leaders, and scholars who fully acknowledge the range of the stigma, needs to be involved to reverse this phenomenon. In addition, governmental and nongovernmental organizations, civil society, interested in the future of our society need to have the appropriate support for their valuable effort of eliminating the stigma

1.10 Research Hypotheses

Considering the description of the situation, the following assumptions are made:

- Following the current HIV prevention and treatment landscape, HIV-positive MSM who have no medical follow-up suffer from increased mortality and morbidity and infect not only men but also women in bisexual relationships. As a result, the inability to engage and help them to behave responsibly leads to missed opportunities to provide adequate care.

- Confidence in healthcare providers remains low. Therefore, these same facilities are considered as threats by MSM due to perceived and experienced stigma.

- Medical education in Haiti does not consider the social and anthropological aspects of specific groups, such as MSM, and the state of research remains very nuclear.

- The community, due to religious and cultural factors, shows intolerance to PLHIV and MSM living with HIV.

1.11 Research Questions

In order to test the hypothesis, the book is driven by these research questions:

Main question:

- How to ensure stigma reduction and proper engagement, adherence and retention along the continuum of HIV services for MSM?

Sub-questions:

- How perceived, enacted and experienced stigma affect the steps of the continuum of HIV services for MSM?

- What are the attitudes of caregivers regarding MSM living with HIV?

- How do the underlying mechanisms of stigma reduction interventions among MSM work?

- What is the proportion of MSM LTFU in each step of the continuum?

- What are the underlying mechanisms and pathways to engagement, adherence and retention along the continuum of HIV services?

1.12 book Objectives

The description of the problem makes it possible to see the daily challenges faced by MSM living with and at risk for HIV in Haiti. The rights and freedom of MSM living with HIV are compromised not only in regards to their sexual orientation but also because they carry the HIV virus. Doubly victims, they have been further oppressed by the new law prohibiting their marriage and promoting activities in their favor. Analyzing the continuum of HIV services for MSM will allow us to embrace the foundation, specific forms and layers of stigma in order to identify, develop and test appropriate mitigation interventions.

Stages of the continuum of services are essential for monitoring and evaluation. Achieving undetectable viral load is the key to improve PLHIV's quality of life and reduce transmission to their partners. In addition, this research helped in developing new knowledge, and reinforced existing one related to this topic. Although MSM are a hard-to-reach community, an outreach and information system with their peers who joined the program helped in enrollment and allowed them to actively participate in the organization of this research. Due to unforeseen circumstances related to political and social unrest in Haiti, various modifications of the initial protocol took place in order to adapt the activities regarding the objectives.

Main objective
- To analyze the impact of stigma on the continuum of HIV services for MSM in order to ascertain why, how and under which circumstances MSM are engaged, linked and retained along the care continuum.

Specific objectives
- To assess the impact of perceived, enacted and experienced on the steps of the continuum of HIV services for MSM.
- To explore the attitudes of caregivers regarding MSM living with HIV
- To analyze the underlying mechanisms of stigma reduction interventions for MSM
- To identify the proportions and the socio-demographic and clinical profiles of the MSM who have left the continuum while exploring the context.
- To generate the underlying mechanisms and pathways for engagement, adherence and retention along the continuum of HIV services for MSM.

1.13 References

1.   Joint United Nations Program on HIV and AIDS. Latest statistics on the status of the AIDS epidemic. Available at: http://www.unaids.org/sites/default/files/media_asset/UNAIDS_FactSheet_en.pdf. (Accessed: 13th March 2021)

2.   Berg, R. C. & Ross, M. W. The Second Closet: A Qualitative Study of HIV Stigma Among Seropositive Gay Men in a Southern U.S. City. *International Journal of Sexual Health* **26,** 186–199 (2014).

3.   Lebouché, B. & Levy, J. J. Nouveaux traitements et indétectabilité du VIH. Un risque dans la relation médecin-patient ? *Médecine et Maladies Infectieuses* **39,** (2009).

4.   Goffman, E. & Kihm, A. *Stigmate: les usages sociaux des handicaps.* (Les Éditions de minuit, 2015).

5.   Progress report 2016: prevent HIV, test and treat all: WHO support for country impact. *World Health Organization*(1970). Available at: https://apps.who.int/iris/handle/10665/251713. (Accessed: 13th March 2021)

6.   Mahajan, A. P. *et al.* Stigma in the HIV/AIDS epidemic: a review of the literature and recommendations for the way forward. *AIDS* **22,** (2008).

7.   Smit, P. J. *et al.* HIV-related stigma within communities of gay men: a literature review. *AIDS Care* **24,** 405–412 (2011).

8.   Amirkhanian, Y. A. Social Networks, Sexual Networks and HIV Risk in Men Who Have Sex with Men. *Current HIV/AIDS Reports* **11,** 81–92 (2014).

9.   Cáceres, C. F. HIV among gay and other men who have sex with men in Latin America and the Caribbean: a hidden epidemic?*. *AIDS* **16,** (2002).

10.   Dramé, F. M., Crawford, E. E., Diouf, D., Beyrer, C. & Baral, S. D. A pilot cohort study to assess the feasibility of HIV prevention science research among men who have sex with men in Dakar, Senegal. *Journal of the International AIDS Society* **16,** 18753 (2013).

11.   Muzyamba, C., Broaddus, E. & Campbell, C. "You cannot eat rights": a qualitative study of views by Zambian HIV-vulnerable women, youth and MSM on

human rights as public health tools. *BMC International Health and Human Rights* **15,** (2015).

12.   Cloete, A., Simbayi, L. C., Kalichman, S. C., Strebel, A. & Henda, N. Stigma and discrimination experiences of HIV-positive men who have sex with men in Cape Town, South Africa. *AIDS Care* **20,** 1105–1110 (2008).

13.   Fay, H. *et al.* Stigma, Health Care Access, and HIV Knowledge Among Men Who Have Sex With Men in Malawi, Namibia, and Botswana. *AIDS and Behavior* **15,** 1088–1097 (2010).

14.   Baral, S., Sifakis, F., Cleghorn, F. & Beyrer, C. Elevated Risk for HIV Infection among Men Who Have Sex with Men in Low- and Middle-Income Countries 2000–2006: A Systematic Review. *PLoS Medicine* **4,** (2007).

15.   Kushwaha, S. *et al.* "But the moment they find out that you are MSM…": a qualitative investigation of HIV prevention experiences among men who have sex with men (MSM) in Ghana's health care system. *BMC Public Health* **17,**(2017).

16.   Link, B. G. & Phelan, J. C. Conceptualizing Stigma. *Annual Review of Sociology* **27,** 363–385 (2001).

17.   Parker, R. & Aggleton, P. HIV and AIDS-related stigma and discrimination: a conceptual framework and implications for action. *Social Science & Medicine* **57,** 13–24 (2003).

18.   Stuber, J., Galea, S. & Link, B. G. Smoking and the emergence of a stigmatized social status. *Social Science & Medicine* *67,* 420–430 (2008).

19.   Beyrer, C. *et al.* A call to action for comprehensive HIV services for men who have sex with men. *The Lancet* **380,** 424–438 (2012).

20.   Risher, K. *et al.* Sexual stigma and discrimination as barriers to seeking appropriate healthcare among men who have sex with men in Swaziland. *Journal of the International AIDS Society* **16,** 18715 (2013).

21.   Horton, R. & Beyrer, C. The Lancet 2012 special theme series: Men who have sex with men and HIV. *PsycEXTRA Dataset* (2012).

22.   International, S.-N. UNAIDS' Global HIV & AIDS statistics 2019 fact sheet. *Share* (2019). Available at: https://share-netinternational.org/unaids-global-hiv-aids-statistics-2019-fact-sheet/. (Accessed: 13th March 2021)

23.   Beyrer, C. *et al.* Global epidemiology of HIV infection in men who have sex with men. *The Lancet* **380,** 367–377 (2012).

24.   Ayala, G. *et al.* Access to Basic HIV-Related Services and PrEP Acceptability among Men Who Have sex with Men Worldwide: Barriers, Facilitators, and Implications for Combination Prevention. *Journal of Sexually Transmitted Diseases* **2013,** 1–11 (2013).

25.   Laptiste, C., Beharry, V. & Edwards-Wescott, P. A review of the response to HIV/AIDS in Trinidad and Tobago: 1983–2010. *SAHARA-J: Journal of Social Aspects of HIV/AIDS* **10,** 72–82 (2013).

26.   Gilman, S. L. AIDS and Syphilis: The Iconography of Disease. *October* **43,** 87 (1987).

26.   HIV/AIDS. *World Health Organization* Available at: https://www.who.int/news-room/fact-sheets/detail/hiv-aids. (Accessed: 13th March 2021)

27.   Beck, EJ. *et al.* Attitudes towards Key Populations in Three Fast Track Caribbean Countries: Haiti, Jamaica and the Dominican Republic. *Journal of HIV and AIDS* **4,** (2018).

28.   MacLean, R. Resources to address stigma related to sexuality, substance use and sexually transmitted and blood-borne infections. *Canada Communicable Disease Report* **44,** 62–67 (2018).

29.   Baxter, C. The Dilemma of Difference: A Multidisciplinary View of Stigma. *Disability, Handicap & Society* **2,** 298–300 (1987).

30.   Seeman, M. & Goffman, E. Stigma: Notes on the Management of Spoiled Identity. *American Sociological Review* **29,** 770 (1964).

31.   Shi, J. *et al.* Assessing the stigma toward chronic carriers of hepatitis B virus: development and validation of a Chinese college students' stigma scale. *Journal of Applied Social Psychology* **43,** 46-55, (2013).

32.   Jacoby, A. Felt versus enacted stigma: A concept revisited. *Social Science & Medicine* **38,** 269–274 (1994).

33.   Scambler, G. Re-framing Stigma: Felt and Enacted Stigma and Challenges to the Sociology of Chronic and Disabling Conditions. *Social Theory & Health* **2,** 29–46

(2004).

34.   Fitzgerald-Husek, A. *et al.* Measuring stigma affecting sex workers (SW) and men who have sex with men (MSM): A systematic review. *PLOS ONE* **12,** (2017).

35.   Winskell, K. & Sabben, G. Sexual stigma and symbolic violence experienced, enacted, and counteracted in young Africans' writing about same-sex attraction. *Social Science & Medicine* **161,** 143–150 (2016).

36.   Earnshaw, V. A. & Chaudoir, S. R. From Conceptualizing to Measuring HIV Stigma: A Review of HIV Stigma Mechanism Measures. *AIDS and Behavior* **13,** (2009).

37.   Earnshaw, V. A., Smith, L. R., Chaudoir, S. R., Amico, K. R. & Copenhaver, M. M. HIV Stigma Mechanisms and Well-Being Among PLWH: A Test of the HIV Stigma Framework. *AIDS and Behavior* **17,** 1785–1795 (2013).

38.   Weiss, M. G., Ramakrishna, J. & Somma, D. Health-related stigma: Rethinking concepts and interventions 1. *Psychology, Health & Medicine* **11,** 277–287 (2006).

39.   Valdiserri RO. HIV/AIDS stigma: an impediment to public health. Am J Public Health. 2002;92: 341–342.

40. Arachu Castro and Paul Farmer, 2005: Understanding and addressing AIDS-related stigma: From Antrhopological Theory to Clinical Practice in Haiti, American Journal of Public Health 95, 53_59.

41. Goffman E. Asylums: Essays on the Social Situation of Mental Patients and Other Inmates. Garden City, NY: Anchor Books; 1961.

42. Tuke DH. The Cagots. J Anthropol Instit Great Britain Ireland. 1880;9:376–385.

43. Fitzgerald-Husek A, Van Wert MJ, Ewing WF, Grosso AL, Holland CE, Katterl R, et al. (2017) Measuring stigma affecting sex workers (SW) and men who have sex with men (MSM): A systematic review. PLoS ONE 12(11): e0188393.

44. Parker R, Aggleton P. HIV and AIDS-related stigma and discrimination: a conceptual framework and implications for action. Soc Sci Med. 2003;57:13–24.

45. Berger BE, Ferrans CE, Lashley FR. Measuring stigma in people with HIV: psychometric assessment of the HIV stigma scale. Res Nurs Health. 2001;24(6):518–29.

46. Swendeman, Dallas & Rotheram-Borus, Mary & Comulada, Warren & Weiss, Robert & Ramos, Maria. (2006). Predictors of HIV-related Stigma among Young People Living with HIV. Health psychology : official journal of the Division of

Health Psychology, American Psychological Association. 25. 501-9. 10.1037/0278-6133.25.4.501.

47. Radcliffe J, Doty N, Hawkins LA, Gaskins CS, Beidas R, Rudy BJ. Stigma and sexual health risk in HIV-positive African American young men who have sex with men. AIDS Patient Care STDS. 2010 Aug;24(8):493-9.

48. Mavhu, W., Willis, N., Mufuka, J. et al. Evaluating a multi-component, community-based program to improve adherence and retention in care among adolescents living with HIV in Zimbabwe: study protocol for a cluster randomized controlled trial. Trials 18, 478 (2017).

49. Zhao Q, Li X, Zhao G, Zhao J, Fang X, Lin X, Stanton B. AIDS knowledge and HIV stigma among children affected by HIV/AIDS in rural China. AIDS Educ Prev. 2011 Aug;23(4):341-50.

50. Klein H, Washington TA. The Pre-Exposure Prophylaxis (PrEP) Stigma Scale: Preliminary findings from a pilot study. *Int Public Health J.* 2019;11(2):185-195.

51. Delany-Moretlwe, S. *et al.* Providing comprehensive health services for young key populations: needs, barriers and gaps. *Journal of the International AIDS Society* **18,** 19833 (2015).

52. Hunt, J., Bristowe, K., Chidyamatare, S. & Harding, R. 'They will be afraid to touch you': LGBTI people and sex workers' experiences of accessing healthcare in Zimbabwe—an in-depth qualitative study. *BMJ Global Health* **2,**(2017).

53. Earnshaw, V. A. & Kalichman, S. C. Stigma Experienced by People Living with HIV/AIDS. *Stigma, Discrimination and Living with HIV/AIDS* 23–38 (2013).

54. Sara Shamos, K. A. H. Men's and Women's Experiences With HIV and Stigma in Swaziland - Sara Shamos, Kari A. Hartwig, Nomsa Zindela. *SAGE Journals* **11,** 277–287 (2009)

55. Ruiseñor-Escudero, H. *et al.* Using a social ecological framework to characterize the correlates of HIV among men who have sex with men in Lomé, Togo. *AIDS Care* **29,** 1169–1177 (2017).

56. Bang on, T. & Supattra, S. Societal awareness of stigma and discrimination against persons living with Human Immunodeficiency Virus (HIV) (PLHIV): Experience of clinicians, PLHIV, general population, and persons who are vulnerable to HIV. *Journal of AIDS and HIV Research* **8,** 25–37 (2016).

57. Castro, A. & Farmer, P. Understanding and Addressing AIDS-Related Stigma: From Anthropological Theory to Clinical Practice in Haiti. *American Journal of Public Health* **95,** 53–59 (2005).

58. Turan, B. *et al.* Framing Mechanisms Linking HIV-Related Stigma, Adherence to Treatment, and Health Outcomes. *American Journal of Public Health* **107,** 863–869 (2017).

59. MacCarthy, S., Brignol, S., Reddy, M., Nunn, A. & Dourado, I. Making the invisible, visible: a cross-sectional study of late presentation to HIV/AIDS services among men who have sex with men from a large urban center of Brazil. *BMC Public Health* **14,** (2014).

60. Judgeo, N. & Moalusi, K. P. My secret: The social meaning of HIV/AIDS stigma. *SAHARA-J: Journal of Social Aspects of HIV/AIDS* **11,** 76–83 (2014).

61. Agozino, B. Drug and Alcohol Consumption and Trade and HIV in the Caribbean: A Review of the Literature. *Journal of HIV/AIDS and Infectious Diseases* 1–12 (2014).

62. Hladik, W. *et al.* Men Who Have Sex with Men in Kampala, Uganda: Results from a Bio-Behavioral Respondent Driven Sampling Survey. *AIDS and Behavior* **21,** 1478–1490 (2016).

63. Multidimensional progress: well-being beyond income. *Social Protection and Human Rights* (2017). Available at: https://socialprotection-humanrights.org/resource/multidimensional-progress-well-beyond-income/. (Accessed: 13th March 2021)

64. Rouzier, V. *et al.* Factors impacting the provision of antiretroviral therapy to people living with HIV: the view from Haiti. *Antiviral Therapy* **19,** 91–104 (2014).

65. Dunbar, W., Pape, J. W. & Coppieters, Y. HIV among men who have sex with men in the Caribbean: reaching the left behind. *Revista Panamericana de Salud Pública* **45,** 1 (2021).

66. Farmer, P. *et al.* Meeting Cholera's Challenge to Haiti and the World: A Joint Statement on Cholera Prevention and Care. *PLoS Neglected Tropical Diseases* **5,** (2011).

67. Walton, D. A. & Ivers, L. C. Responding to Cholera in Post-Earthquake Haiti. *New England Journal of Medicine* **364,** 3–5 (2011).

68. Koenig, S. *et al.* Successes and challenges of HIV treatment programs in Haiti: aftermath of the earthquake. *HIV Therapy* **4,** 145–160 (2010).

69. Daniels, J. P. Haiti's complex history with HIV, and recent successes. *The Lancet HIV* **6,** (2019).

70. Lowrance, D. W. *et al.* Public Health Progress in Haiti. *The American Journal of Tropical Medicine and Hygiene* **97,** 1–3 (2017).

71. Jean Louis, F. *et al.* Building and Rebuilding: The National Public Health Laboratory Systems and Services Before and After the Earthquake and Cholera Epidemic, Haiti, 2009–2015. *The American Journal of Tropical Medicine and Hygiene* **97,** 21–27 (2017).

72. Kinsler, J. J., Wong, M. D., Sayles, J. N., Davis, C. & Cunningham, W. E. The Effect of Perceived Stigma from a Health Care Provider on Access to Care Among a Low-Income HIV-Positive Population. *AIDS Patient Care and STDs* **21,** 584–592 (2007).

73. The 2016 United Nations Political Declaration on Ending AIDS sets the world on the Fast-Track to end the epidemic by 2030. *UNAIDS, 2016 United Nations Political Declaration on Ending AIDS sets world on the FastTrack to end the epidemic by 2030 Comments* Available at: https://unaids.org.vn/2016-united-nations-political-declaration-ending-aids-sets-world-fast-track-end-epidemic-2030/. (Accessed: 13th March 2021)

74. Haiti Country Operational Plan (COP) 2019 Strategic ... Available at: https://www.state.gov/wp-content/uploads/2019/09/Haiti_COP19-Strategic-Directional-Summary_public.pdf. (Accessed: 13th March 2021)

75. Bulletin de Surveillance Épidémiologique VIH/Sida no 19 ... Available at: https://reliefweb.int/sites/reliefweb.int/files/resources/Bulletin%20de%20Surveillance%20%20%20Epidemiologique%20VIHSida%20no%2019%2C%20decembre%202018.pdf. (Accessed: 13th March 2021)

76. Christopoulos, K. A., Das, M. & Colfax, G. N. Linkage and Retention in HIV Care among Men Who Have Sex with Men in the United States. *Clinical Infectious Diseases* **52,** (2011).

77. Évaluation de la Prestation des Services de Soins de Santé en Haïti... Available at: https://www.dhsprogram.com/pubs/pdf/SR211/SR211.pdf. (Accessed: 13th March 2021)

78. Research for universal health coverage: World health report 2013. *World Health Organization* Available at:

https://www.who.int/publications/i/item/9789240690837. (Accessed: 13th March 2021)

79. Perry, H. *et al.* Long-Term Reductions in Mortality Among Children Under Age 5 in Rural Haiti: Effects of a Comprehensive Health System in an Impoverished Setting. *American Journal of Public Health* **97,** 240–246 (2007).

80. Dowell, S. F., Tappero, J. W. & Frieden, T. R. Public Health in Haiti — Challenges and Progress. *New England Journal of Medicine* **364,** 300–301 (2011).

81. Stangl, A. L., Lloyd, J. K., Brady, L. M., Holland, C. E. & Baral, S. A systematic review of interventions to reduce HIV-related stigma and discrimination from 2002 to 2013: how far have we come? *Journal of the International AIDS Society* **16,** 18734 (2013).

82. Smith, A. M. Associations between the sexual behaviour of men who have sex with men and the structure and composition of their social networks. *Sexually Transmitted Infections* **80,** 455–458 (2004).

83. Beyrer, C. *et al.* The Expanding Epidemics of HIV Type 1 Among Men Who Have Sex With Men in Low- and Middle-Income Countries: Diversity and Consistency. *Epidemiologic Reviews* **32,** 137–151 (2010).

84. Programmatic Mapping and Size Estimation of Key Populations in Haiti. *FHI360* Available at: https://www.fhi360.org/sites/default/files/media/documents/resource-linkages-haiti-size-key-populations-april-2017.pdf. (Accessed: 13th March 2021)

85. Oldenburg, C. E. Integrated HIV prevention and care for key populations. *The Lancet HIV* **6,** (2019).

86. HIV prevalence among FSWs and MSM in Haiti. Available at: https://www.paho.org/hq/index.php?option=com_docman&view=download&category_slug=vigilancia-poblaciones-clave-4737&alias=19315-haiti-vigilancia-epidemiologica-vih-315&Itemid=270&lang=en. (Accessed: 13th March 2021)

87. Risher, K., Mayer, K. H. & Beyrer, C. HIV treatment cascade in MSM, people who inject drugs, and sex workers. *Current Opinion in HIV and AIDS* **10,** 420–429 (2015).

88. Tudrej, B. V. La responsabilité sociale des facultés de médecine, un moyen de réconcilier les étudiants avec leur engagement médical. *Pédagogie Médicale* **14,** 73–74 (2013).

89. Boelen, C. Coordinating medical education and health care systems: the power of the social accountability approach. *Medical Education* **52,** 96–102 (2017).

90. Boelen, C. & Woollard, B. Social accountability and accreditation: a new frontier for educational institutions. *Medical Education* **43,** 887–894 (2009).

91. Consensus mondial sur la responsabilité sociale des facultés de médecine. *Pédagogie Médicale* **12,** 37–48 (2011).

92. ang X, Li X, Qiao S, Li L, Parker C, Shen Z, Zhou Y. Intersectional stigma and psychosocial well-being among MSM living with HIV in Guangxi, China. AIDS Care. 2020 May;32(sup2):5-13. doi: 10.1080/09540121.2020.1739205. Epub 2020 Mar 10. PMID: 32156159; PMCID: PMC7172016.

93. Alexandra Marshall S, Brewington KM, Kathryn Allison M, Haynes TF, Zaller ND. Measuring HIV-related stigma among healthcare providers: a systematic review. AIDS Care. 2017 Nov;29(11):1337-1345. doi: 10.1080/09540121.2017.1338654. Epub 2017 Jun 9. PMID: 28599599.

94. Dubov A, Galbo P Jr, Altice FL, Fraenkel L. Stigma and Shame Experiences by MSM Who Take PrEP for HIV Prevention: A Qualitative Study. Am J Mens Health. 2018 Nov;12(6):1843-1854. doi: 10.1177/1557988318797437. Epub 2018 Aug 30. PMID: 30160195; PMCID: PMC6199453.

PART 2. METHODS

2.1 Conceptual Framework: Realist Methodology

Guided by a realist approach, through this book we took the continuum of HIV services for MSM, a theory-based intervention, and set out to explore the contexts and elicit the mechanisms behind the outcomes (1). Finally, we make key recommendations for capacity building, improvement and sustainable impact.

"The term 'realist evaluation' is drawn from Pawson and Tilley's seminal work, *Realistic Evaluation* (1997) (2). It is a member of the family of theory-based evaluation approaches. Theory-based evaluation starts by clarifying the 'programme theory' – that is, clarifying how programme activities are understood to cause (or contribute to) outcomes and impacts. What distinguishes realist evaluation from other forms of theory-based evaluation are the particular assumptions that realist philosophy makes about the nature of reality, how causation works, and what these assumptions imply for evaluation design, methods and utilization" (3–5).

"Realist approaches assume that nothing works everywhere or for everyone, and that context really does make a difference to programme outcomes (6,7). Consequently, policy-makers and practitioners need to understand how and why programmes work and don't work in different contexts, so that they are better equipped to make decisions about which programmes or policies to use and how to adapt them to local contexts" (8-10).

The contexts' exploration began with a deep understanding of the contexts, not only in Haïti, but in other similar settings as well. We started by searching the epidemiology, social and cultural factors driving the HIV epidemic among MSM in the Caribbean region, highlighting the regional and national responses, and assessing what remains to be addressed to close the gaps in order to end AIDS by 2030. Then, we reviewed the literature to examine what is known about stigma and discrimination among MSM living with and at risk for HIV, what is the impact of stigma on the steps of continuum and what interventions and/or programs have been developed to address the problem. Finally, we explored the Haitian socio-medical and cultural contexts to study the attitudes that medical students in Haiti harbour toward MSM living with HIV in order to better understand how stigma and other factors may impair healthcare, and to explore suggestions of opportunities in line with the values of social accountability. We chose to focus on medical students because they represent the next generation of clinicians responsible for HIV care efforts and they often reflect attitudes held in their society and community of practice.

In eliciting the mechanisms, we set out the epistemological framework of a realist approach to introduce the context-mechanism-outcome (CMO) relationships as a key analytical tool in a systematic review and a program evaluation. With the systematic review, we highlighted the mechanisms through which stigma mitigation interventions generate better HIV prevention and contribute to the continuum for MSM. We reviewed international program frameworks and scientific publications from tested interventions regarding specific contexts. The realist evaluation assessed the continuum of HIV services for MSM in Haiti. We developed the initial program theory based on participant observations, discussions with key informants and program frameworks review. Second, we tested the program theory using a mixed-method explanatory design study. Then, the initial program theory was refined by eliciting the mechanisms and pathways to improve the continuum.

Finally, converted into strategies, we listed the mechanisms and pathways based on a comprehensive classification: intrapersonal, interpersonal, health systems-based and structural.

Realist Evaluation can be represented at four levels with regard to the continuum. On the level of philosophy, realist evaluation is grounded in realism and in systems theory, which is the foundation of the linkages across the continuum. Realist evaluation itself is a particular evaluation theory, which we explored by reviewing frameworks and conducting key informants' interviews and participant observations. Realist Evaluation develops a particular kind of program theory, structured as Context- Mechanism- Outcome Configuration (CMOC), which we constructed through the systematic review and the evaluation. Lastly, substantive theory feeds realist evaluation with clues on the mechanisms through which programs work and the contexts in which they will work (4-7).

As presented in figure 1 below, in responding to the need of stigma mitigation, engagement and retention, various intervention components have been developed to produce the desired outcomes. However, seamless and dynamic interactions are present among interventions, contexts, mechanisms and outcomes. Interventions don't produce outcomes in a linear way. Thus, the methodology is built to analyse the intervention and the outcomes while identifying the contextual factors and generating the mechanisms for overall improvement.

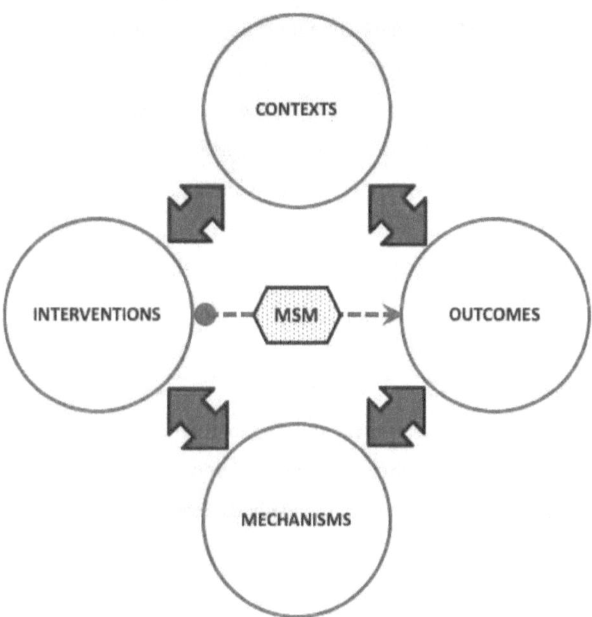

Figure 1. Interactions among interventions, contexts, mechanisms and outcomes.

With regard to evaluation, the assumptions about reality mean that programs and policies are real and can have real effects - positive, negative, intended and unintended. Social programs operate as open systems in which all levels are interacting. Program change systems and systems change programs. This means that evaluation is not simple and outcomes are not linear. There are always multiple and competing mechanisms operating. Mechanisms also interact with their context, which is why a program can generate 'x' outcomes in one setting and 'y' outcomes in another (3,4,5-7).

Realist evaluation begins with the formulation of a theory behind the development of an intervention, known as initial program theory (IPT). IPT is formulated on the basis of a review of literature and documents and/or the experience of stakeholders involved in the intervention, and describes how the intervention is supposed to generate change (3). Our IPTs for the realist review and the realist evaluation were developed from participant observations at the health facilities, discussions with the program coordinators, healthcare providers and MSM and, review of program frameworks and reports. The basis of the program theory consists of a context-mechanism-outcome configuration, which describes patterns or causal chains: certain components of the intervention trigger certain mechanisms within individuals (or groups of individuals) that produce certain outcomes. IPT is then tested through empirical research where the intervention has been implemented. In our cases, data were collected through literature review and a mixed method explanatory design. The analysis of data in these cases served to refine the preliminary IPT. Realist evaluation provides a deeper understanding of the links between the program and the outcomes by exploring the interactions between program, actors, context and mechanisms, and consequently offers results that can be acted upon by decision makers (1,2,5,6).

2.2 Overall Methodology of the book

The overall methodology applied, presented in figure 3, allowed us to describe the contexts, generating the mechanisms and enabling the outcomes through a thoughtful succession of steps from literature reviews, qualitative and mixed methods explanatory researches.

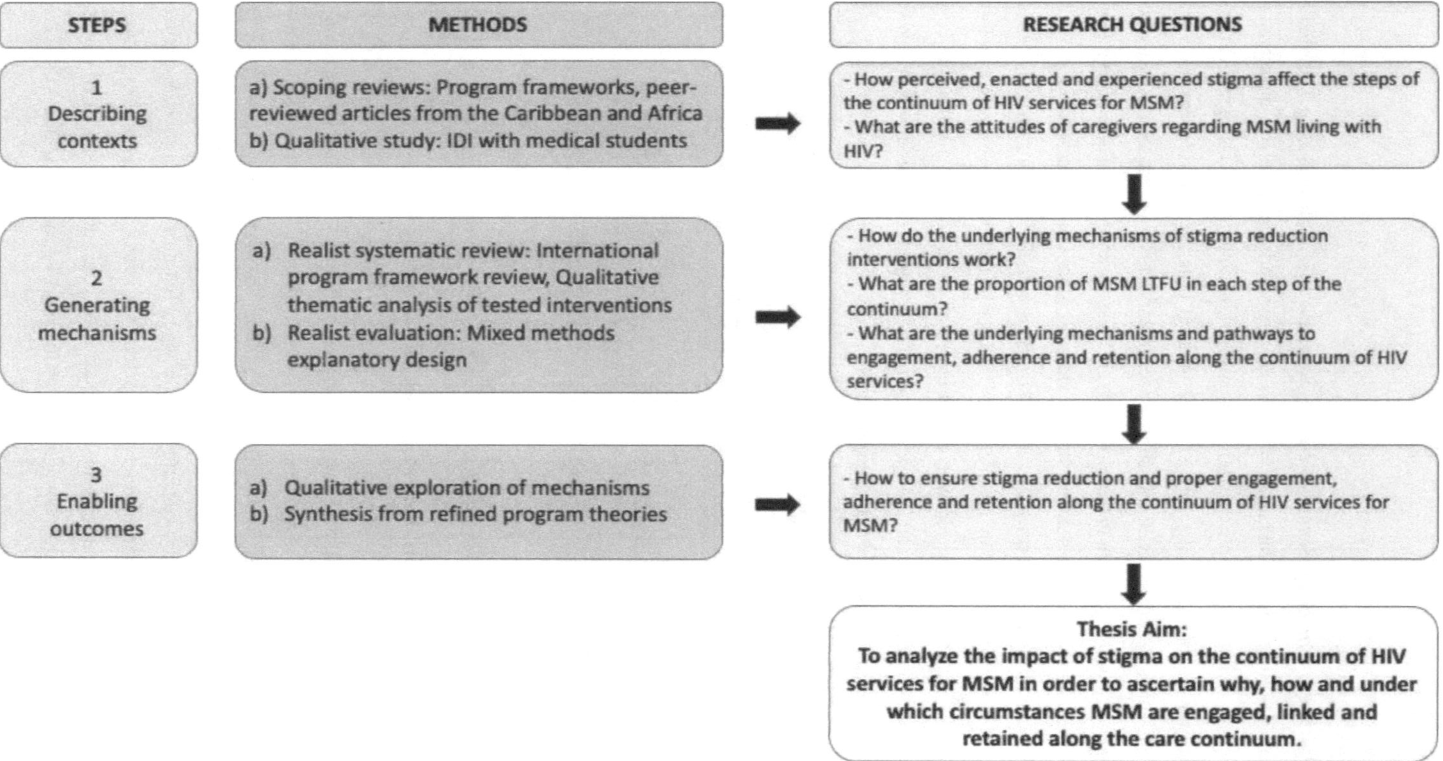

Figure 2. Methodology outline: Context – Mechanism – Outcome (CMO) configuration of the book processes and designs

2.3 Research Settings

- ***Quisqueya University School of Health Sciences:*** It is a medical school located in Port-au-Prince, the capital city of Haiti. As the largest private university, the school of Health Sciences comprises 800 students originating from all administrative departments of the country. The six-year medical program is divided into two-year basic sciences and four-year clinical sciences in partnership with associated academic hospitals located not only in the capital city, but also in several rural and urban regions of the country ensuring practice through various cultures and contexts. The program also entails clinical placements in infectious diseases and HIV settings where students work under the supervision of clinical tutors. As part of the social accountability reform process for accreditation renewal, efforts are being made to have a substantial basic science, clinical, and epidemiological community-oriented research activity within the university and associated academic hospitals.

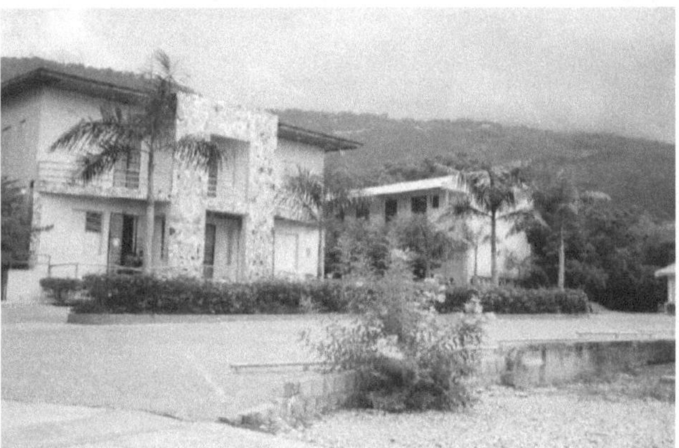

Figure 3. Quisqueya University, Port-au-Prince, Haïti. (Source: UniQ)

- ***GHESKIO centers:*** GHESKIO works collaboratively with the Haitian Government to implement the prevention and care model to a network of 27 hospitals and healthcare centers throughout the country through training, monitoring and evaluation. The linkage program aims to deliver and optimize services that reduce HIV transmission among MSM and their sexual partners and extend life for those who are HIV-positive. This seamless integration of interventions requires strong linkages among program elements so that HIV transmission is reduced and people diagnosed with HIV obtain early access to services, including ART. This model necessitates that MSM flow efficiently, consistently, and sustainably through the entire HIV continuum of prevention, care, and treatment services.

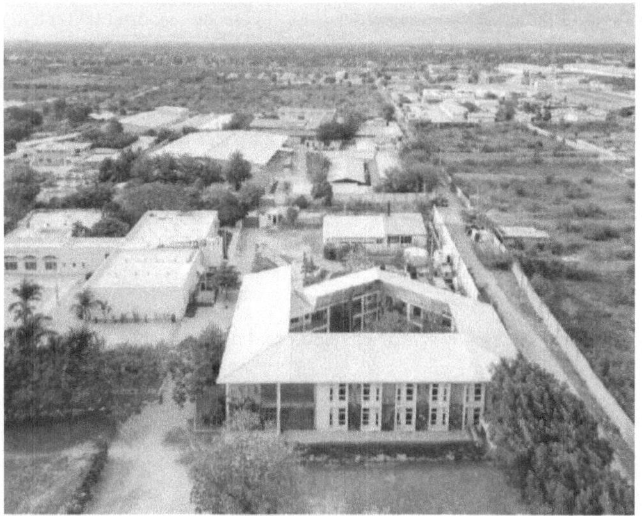

Figure 4. GHESKIO centers, Port-au-Prince, Haïti (Source: GHESKIO)

2.4 Research Participants

- *Medical students:* for the qualitative study, we used purposive sampling to select the research participants which comprised 11 males and 11 females. Ages of the participants vary from 23 to 26 years; 20 of them identified themselves as Christians (Catholic and Protestants) and 2 did not mention their religion. The participants were in their final step of the clinical sciences program and already spent three years in clinical placement at the associated academic hospitals.

- *MSM:* MSM were active and non-active patients from GHESKIO's cohort. We also conducted several interviews and informal conversations with MSM networks' members in Port-au-Prince. To build the cohort, a retrospective review of MSM living with HIV electronic medical records (EMR) was used to collect data using a standardized excel form. As an exploratory part in nature no formal sample size calculations were conducted. We used the EMR system to review all files and select MSM living with HIV patients aged 18 years and above and enrolled between January 2017 and December 2018 were screened for eligibility to be included in the study.

MSM were defined as men who reported sex with another man either at enrolment or subsequently during follow-up. Patient files were excluded if they missed data on important variables including date for start of care, sexual orientation and age.

- ***Key informants:*** The key informants involved linkages program coordinators, policy makers, program evaluators, monitoring and evaluation officers, sites technical coordinators, healthcare givers (doctors and nurses) and MSM peer educators and community health workers.

2.5 Step 1- Describing Contexts

To describe the contexts, two literature reviews and a qualitative study were conducted.

2.5.1 Design and Data Collection

The first scoping review aimed to present: 1) the HIV infection among MSM in term of epidemiology, social and cultural factors driving the epidemic, regional and national responses, and 2) what remains to be addressed to close the gaps in order to identify areas for further research and program development towards ending AIDS by 2030. To identify peer-reviewed articles, abstracts and reports of HIV studies conducted among MSM in the Caribbean we performed a search of PubMed and Scopus, on June 2019, using Medical Subject Headings (MeSH) terms or other associated terms for HIV cross referenced with ''stigma,'' ''discrimination reduction,'' "social stigma," or "homophobia," as well as "men who have sex with men," "gay men," "gay man," "bisexual men," "bisexual man," "homosexual men," "homosexual man," or "Homosexuality, Male", "high-risk groups", "prevalence", "Caribbean", and individual country names. We considered original research articles, reviews and reports published in English, French and Spanish over the period of January 2009 through May 2019. The 2009–2019 period was selected since an emergence of international interest in the role of MSM in HIV epidemics globally has become more apparent and major innovations took place in HIV testing, prevention, treatment, retention strategies, monitoring and evaluation tools and elimination initiatives. The initial screening search was based on the titles and abstracts of the articles. Following the PubMed and Scopus search, we reviewed bibliographies of major articles for further references not indexed in the search engine. We also reviewed relevant documents from international organizations such as UNAIDS, Pan Caribbean Partnership against HIV/AIDS (PANCAP) and AIDS case reporting to the Pan American Health Organization (PAHO)/WHO, studies and reports on the social and cultural aspects of Caribbean homosexuality. For peer-reviewed articles, inclusion criteria were determined a priori to be: studies including HIV prevalence data, sociocultural risk factors driving the epidemic among MSM, description of regional and national efforts and potential challenges and barriers to effective control of the epidemic among MSM; country report or an abstract at a conference with peer-reviewed blinded abstract selection process; studies from Caribbean regions. This report concentrates exclusively on publications relating on MSM living in the Caribbean countries.

The second scoping review aimed to review the published literature to examine what is known about stigma and discrimination of HIV-infected MSM, what is the impact of these issues on the continuum of care and what interventions and/or programs have been developed to address them in two regions in the world: Africa and the Caribbean. In line with the research questions, articles that correlated Stigma, MSM and HIV were identified. The collection period occurred in March and April 2018. Articles published between march 2008 and march 2018 were surveyed. The analysis followed the predetermined eligibility criteria. PubMed search for all published articles pertaining to HIV/AIDS infected MSM related stigma was run. Then the 10-year period and the human species filters were applied. This timeframe of a decade was used to provide sufficient historical perspective on trends in stigma measurement and developed interventions. Each of the abstracts identified was reviewed. Following the PubMed search, bibliographies of major articles for further references not indexed in the search engine were reviewed. The following four criteria had to be met in order to include a study in this review: the study is conducted in Africa or the Caribbean; the study subjects include MSM and include results separately about MSM (either attitudes, behaviours, outcomes about MSM or from MSM); Stigma or discrimination is reported as an exposure or outcome, its relationship to people with HIV or MSM is addressed in the study; the study is about HIV, either its prevention or treatment, access to care, affordability of care, or health care structures related to HIV infected patients. We also included studies that lacked a clear description of the measures used or those that used non-validated measures for stigma. Article citations were organized, uploaded and reviewed using excel spreadsheet. The title, author, journal and year of publication were then exported for title and abstract review. Abstracts were screened to determine whether they included relevant information. If the abstract was deemed compatible, the full article was then retrieved and screened for relevant information. If the full text had to be obtained to determine if the abstract was relevant, the full text was reviewed.

The third study was a qualitative exploration of the attitudes that medical students harbour towards MSM and better understand the extent to which stigma and other factors may impair actual and future healthcare, and secondly, to explore suggestions of opportunities for making such services socially accountable. We utilized a qualitative study design by using a grounded theory approach regarding the context of Haiti (11). We sought to assess the attitudes of medical students towards MSM living with HIV based on an inductive approach, which provided the framework for data analysis. We used purposive sampling to select the research participants which comprised 11 males and 11 females. Ages of the participants vary from 23 to 26 years; 20 of them identified themselves as Christians (Catholic and Protestants) and 2 did not mention their religion. The participants were in their final step of the clinical sciences program and already spent three years in clinical placement at the associated academic hospitals. Among them, 17 indicated that they have already provided care for MSM during their clerkships in HIV facilities. For those who indicated that they had never served any MSM and therefore did not have any experience to share, we asked them to imagine what would happen if they were to take care of MSM. Eligibility was met if they were registered in final year and had clinical training and practice in providing care to PLHIV. In order to ensure maximum variation, we managed to elicit views from diverse categories of students with different ages, sex, city of origin and religious beliefs.

2.5.2 Data Analysis

For the first literature synthesis each article reviewed was analysed with a standardized tool, seeking to identify data on the HIV epidemic among MSM, social and cultural factors, the regional and national responses, the challenges and barriers that remain in the Caribbean. Data were extracted using forms detailing study location, study objectives; thematic areas mentioned above; data collection; methodology (design, setting, population, MSM sample size); results and outcomes; and specific sexual and HIV stigma-related issues. After data extraction for each paper, the studies were grouped and combined with other relevant documents mentioned above according to aims of this review.

For the second review, from each article, data were obtained on: the design of the study, either it was quantitative, qualitative or mixed-method; date of data collection; country of the study; location where data were collected (healthcare setting or community); the main objective; the targets ; the sample size; the type of stigma measured, analysed or mentioned (perceived, enacted or both); the stigma scale used if stigma was measured; the study purpose (description or intervention); the outcomes and the main findings. If any of the data mentioned could not be obtained or was not mentioned, we then classified it as "not specified".

For the qualitative exploration, recorded interviews were transcribed verbatim. We reviewed the transcribed data to ensure understanding and then compared these transcripts with the original audio recordings for accuracy. The primary author read and reviewed the transcripts multiple times and selected one transcript for the initial open coding. To validate the coding process, a clean copy of the same transcript was de-identified and given to another experienced qualitative researcher to conduct a separate independent open coding which was later verified by co-authors. The primary author assessed both coding outputs and came up with one generic coding frame for indexing the rest of the codes. Relationships and comparisons between themes were generated from the coding frame in an iterative process. This ensured that attention was given for consistent patterns within the data focusing on similarities and differences on responses given by participants to aid analysis and interpretation. Our approach to data analysis was based on thematic analysis in line with the study aim.

2.6 Step 2- Eliciting Mechanisms for Outcomes Improvement
To elicit the mechanisms, we carried out a realist review and a realist evaluation of the linkages program.

2.6.1 Development of the IPT
In the systematic review, first, we developed a preliminary model to identify how context influences mechanisms to generate outcomes. We conducted a scoping review of the grey literature and international program frameworks from the United States Agency for International Development (USAID), the U.S. President's Emergency Plan for AIDS Relief (PEPFAR) and the LINKAGES project. Then, the preliminary model is refined based on a systematic review of the literature to investigate whether, why, or how intervention strategies produce observed outcomes, and in what circumstances. We reviewed the international program frameworks to develop a preliminary model on stigma reduction interventions for HIV prevention and care outcomes. To test our preliminary model we performed a systematic search of Pub Med and SCOPUS, on March 2019, using MESH terms or other associated terms for HIV cross referenced with ''stigma,'' ''discrimination reduction,'' "social stigma," or "homophobia," as well as "men who have sex with men," "gay men," "gay man," "bisexual men," "bisexual man," "homosexual men," "homosexual man," or "Homosexuality, Male."

Our first screening included studies that described an empirical evaluation of the efficacy or effectiveness of intervention to reduce stigma related to MSM or HIV. Inclusion criteria included: presentation of interventions' evaluation, clear description of the sampling methods, and stigma mitigation related to MSM or HIV infection as a primary or secondary outcome. Selected qualitative, quantitative and mixed methods intervention studies from all countries were included. We included ancestry searches of the articles included in the first screening using the same inclusion criteria.

For the realist evaluation, we explored the development of the continuum by participant observations at the health facilities, discussions with the program coordinators, healthcare providers and MSM and, review of program frameworks and reports. Guided by realist evaluation principles, the findings were analysed thematically. This IPT served as a hypothesis that was tested through a mixed methods design.

2.6.2 Testing of the IPT

For the realist review, standardized excel forms were piloted and used for data abstraction. Data were abstracted by two reviewers for each included study using the developed standardized form. The data abstraction form included information about date of data collection, country of study, study aim, intervention strategies, target population, sample size of MSM participants, measured outcomes as defined by the study team (HIV stigma, sexual stigma or both), what form of stigma was addressed by the intervention, whether/how stigma was measured in the study population and the underlined structural factors. Data analysis was conducted qualitatively after extraction. Codes and themes were generated in regards to the context, mechanisms, and intervention strategies. In an iterative way, we followed the process to have the initial model and refine it.

For the realist evaluation, for this second step, we carried out a mixed methodology with a sequential explanatory design (10-12). Often used by realist research in health, this design allowed to evaluate the continuum in two phases: a quantitative phase to build the continuum from a cross-sectional analysis, and a qualitative phase was then initiated to explore the motivators and facilitators related to linkage along the continuum. Recorded interviews were transcribed verbatim. Our inductive approach to data analysis was based on the thematic analysis in line with the study aim. The methods were integrated through triangulation of quantitative and qualitative results

2.6.3 Refining the Program Theory Through Mechanisms Identification

Refining the program theory through mechanisms identification: the aim of this step was to inductively develop and extract themes for classification of qualitatively analysed data into mechanisms and respective pathways using thematic content analysis. The IPT provided a basic framework on understanding how and why mechanisms generate the outcomes. Codes and themes were generated in regard to the context, mechanisms, pathways and intervention strategies in an iterative way. For each outcome, we tested the association with an identified mechanism taking into consideration the context.

2.7 Step 3- Enabling the outcomes

After refining the IPT through mechanisms identification, we exploited the pathways to enable the outcomes to formulate a combination of intervention strategies based on three levels: intrapersonal, interpersonal, health systems based and structural.

2.8 Trustworthiness of the work

Four techniques were used to support the trustworthiness of the qualitative content analysis: credibility, dependability, conformability and transferability (12,13). Prior to data collection and in order to understand the contextual factors relating to the HIV care continuum for MSM, three meetings and two participant observation sessions were held with MSM patients, HIV caregivers and medical students at two HIV-associated academic centers and at the main campus of the Université Quisqueya. Credibility was established by selecting an in-depth interview method for the data collection and by the researcher who conducted the interviews being familiar with the context (14). Dependability was established by describing the data analysis in detail and providing direct citations to reveal the basis from which the analysis was conducted (15). The citations used in this article were translated from Haitian Creole into English with the help of a translator, to maintain accuracy and context as much as possible (16). The conformability and consistency of the analysis were established by holding meetings for the authors to discuss preliminary findings, emerging codes and themes until a consensus was reached. To enhance the transferability of the findings, a description of the context, selection and demographics of participants, data collection and process of analysis is provided to enable the reader determine whether the results of this study are transferable to another context (17).

2.9 Ethics Statement

Ethical approval for the study was obtained from the Haitian Group for the Study of Kaposi's Sarcoma and Opportunistic Infections' human right committee and the Cornell University Weill Medical College's Research Ethics Board. At the level of the program, permission was obtained from the facility managers, and finally, consents from the participants and the key informants were obtained. Confidentiality was assured and pseudonyms were used for all respondents. Prior to interviewing, the study purpose and expectations of involvement were explained in Haitian Creole to the participants. We obtained oral and written informed consent from all participants. Data was stored in a secure place and the anonymity was maintained through de-identification.

2.10 References

1- The Realist Evaluation Paradigm for Practice. *Realist Evaluation in Practice* 22–41 doi:10.4135/9781849209762.

2- Westhorp, G. Understanding Mechanisms in Realist Evaluation and Research. *Doing Realist Research* 41–58 (2018). doi:10.4135/9781526451729.n4

3- Henry, G. T. *Realist evaluation: an emerging theory in support of practice*. (Jossey-Bass Publ., 1998).

4- Qualitatively-Driven Mixed Method Designs. *Mixed Method Design* 85–116 (2016). doi:10.4324/9781315424538-14

5- Moser, A. & Korstjens, I. Series: Practical guidance to qualitative research. Part 1: Introduction. European Journal of General Practice 23, 271–273 (2017).

6- Korstjens, I. & Moser, A. Series: Practical guidance to qualitative research. Part 2: Context, research questions and designs. *European Journal of General Practice* 23, 274–279 (2017).

7- Moser, A. & Korstjens, I. Series: Practical guidance to qualitative research. Part 3: Sampling, data collection and analysis. *European Journal of General Practice* 24, 9–18 (2017).

8- Kaur, M. Application of mixed method approach in public health research. *Indian Journal of Community Medicine* 41, 93 (2016).

9- Pawson, R. & Sridharan, S. Theory-driven evaluation of public health programmes. *Evidence-based Public Health* 43–62 (2009).

10- de Souza, D. E. Elaborating the Context-Mechanism-Outcome configuration (CMOc) in realist evaluation: A critical realist perspective. *Evaluation* 19, 141–154 (2013).

11- Triana, R. Evidence-Based Policy: A Realist Perspective, by Ray Pawson. *Journal of Policy Practice* 7, 321–323 (2008).

12- Pawson, R. & Tilley, N. Realistic Evaluation Bloodlines. *American Journal of Evaluation* 22, 317–324 (2001).

13- Evidence-based policy: a realist perspective. *Making Realism Work* 42–65 (2005).

14- Pawson, R., Greenhalgh, T., Harvey, G. & Walshe, K. Realist review - a new method of systematic review designed for complex policy interventions. *Journal of Health Services Research & Policy* 10, 21–34 (2005).

15- Korstjens, I. & Moser, A. Series: Practical guidance to qualitative research. Part 4: Trustworthiness and publishing. *European Journal of General Practice* 24, 120–124 (2017).

16- Cypress, B. S. Fostering Effective Mentoring Relationships in Qualitative Research. *Dimensions of Critical Care Nursing* 39, 305–311 (2020).

17- Ozawa, S. & Pongpirul, K. 10 best resources on … mixed methods research in health systems. *Health Policy and Planning* 29, 323–327 (2013).

PART 3. RESULTS

WITH RESPECT TO THE REALIST METHODOLOGY APPLIED THROUGH THIS book, THE RESULTS ARE PRESENTED IN TWO STEPS:
STEP 1: DESCRIBING CONTEXTS
STEP 2: ELICITING MECHANISMS FOR OUTCOMES IMPROVEMENT

STEP 1 DESCRIBING CONTEXTS
To describe the contexts, three studies (two literature reviews and a qualitative research) were carried out:

1. The study 1: "HIV among Men who have Sex with Men in the Caribbean: Reaching the left behind" presents the epidemiology, social and cultural factors driving the HIV epidemic among MSM in the Caribbean region and to highlight the regional and national responses, and what remains to be addressed to close the gaps in order to end AIDS by 2030.

2. The study 2: "Impact of Stigma on the continuum of HIV services for Men who have Sex with Men in the Caribbean and Africa" analyzed scientific publications to examine what is known about stigma and discrimination from the perspective of MSM living with, what is the impact of these issues on the continuum of care and what interventions and/or programs have been developed to address stigma. This work is focused on two regions: Africa and the Caribbean.

3. The study 3: "Attitudes of medical students towards men who have sex with men living with HIV: implications for social accountability" explored the attitudes that medical students in Haiti harbour toward Men who have Sex with Men living with HIV in order to better understand how stigma and other factors may impair healthcare, and to explore suggestions of opportunities in line with the values of social accountability.

Presentation of the study 1:

To start the context exploration, this first study presents an overview of the HIV epidemic that hit the Caribbean in the late '70s and it currently reflects the highest HIV seroprevalence rate after sub-Saharan Africa. Men who have Sex with Men (MSM) in the Caribbean, like in other places in the world, have been one of the constituencies most affected by the epidemic, and continue to be vulnerable to high rates of HIV-related morbidity and mortality. Even though high-quality data on prevalence and healthcare services utilization among MSM in several Caribbean countries is limited, gay men and other MSM accounted for nearly a quarter of new infections in 2017. From the social construction of heteronormativity in the region, several social and cultural factors, gender norms, and strong stigma associated with HIV and homosexuality lie behind this high burden. Caribbean cultural constructions of masculinity impose obligations and restrictions leading to risky sexual practices besides the practice of sex between men remains a criminal offence in several Caribbean countries. In term of response, international funding programmes have economically supported the region and have also launched specific initiatives, in partnership with national institutions and civil society organizations to expand MSM's access to and retention in HIV services. But, persistent challenges mainly linked to the conservative nature of Caribbean societies makes it difficult to identify and reach MSM. To end the AIDS epidemic by 2030, the Caribbean and global community urgently need to defy expectations to no longer keep unchecked the invisibility of MSM.

Study 1

HIV among Men who have Sex with Men in the Caribbean: Reaching the left behind Willy Dunbar[1], Jean William Pape[2] and Yves Coppieters[1]

1 Université. libre de Bruxelles (ULB), Brussels, Belgium.

2 Groupe Haitien d'Etude du Sarcome de Kaposi et des Infections Opportunistes (GHESKIO), Port-au-Prince, Haiti

Citation

Dunbar W, Pape JW, Coppieters Y. HIV among men who have sex with men in the Caribbean: reaching the left behind. Rev Panam Salud Publica. 2021;45: e12.

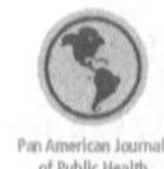

HIV among men who have sex with men in the Caribbean: reaching the left behind

Willy Dunbar[1], Jean William Pape[2] and Yves Coppieters[1]

Suggested citation   Dunbar W, Pape JW, Coppieters Y. HIV among men who have sex with men in the Caribbean: reaching the left behind. Rev
Panam Salud Publica. 2021;45:e12.https://doi.org/10.26633/RPSP.2021.12

Keywords   HIV; sexually transmitted diseases; equity; Caribbean Region.

The HIV epidemic hit the Caribbean in the late '70s, and currently this subregion of the Americas presents the highest HIV seroprevalence rate (1.2%) after sub-Saharan Africa (1). Approximately 340 000 persons are living with HIV/AIDS in the Caribbean. This number includes, in 2018, 16 000 persons who became newly infected. 72.0 % of people living with HIV (PLWHIV) in the Caribbean were aware of their HIV status. Of those who were aware, 77.0 % were accessing antiretroviral treatment (ART). Of those on treatment, 74.0 % were virally suppressed. Nearly 90.0 % of new infections in the Caribbean in 2017 occurred in Cuba, Dominican Republic, Haiti and Jamaica while 87.0 % of deaths from AIDS-related illness occurred in the Dominican Republic, Haiti and Jamaica (1).

Even though the Caribbean countries consider health as a fundamental human right and entitlement, the healthcare systems are meaningfully differentiated from one country to another in terms of healthcare delivery, health policies, financing and governance (2). In term of meeting expectations regarding the HIV epidemic, progress has been made to ensure adherence to care and prevention through awareness, education and pre-exposure prophylaxis (PrEP) (3, 4).

A focus on men who have sex with men (MSM) in the Caribbean showed that they accounted for nearly a quarter of new infections in 2017. Thus, MSM are the group most affected by HIV in the Caribbean (5), and several factors are behind this high burden. Although sex between men is rather frequent in the region, male homosexual behaviour does not usually imply homosexual or bisexual self-identities (6, 7). Homosexuality is still a source of stigma, discrimination and human rights violations in many islands (8). Many MSM fear public exposure,

[1] Université libre de Bruxelles, Brussels, Belgium. ✉ Willy Dunbar, wdunbar@ulb.ac.be

[2] Groupe Haïtien d'Etude du Sarcome de Kaposi et des Infections Opportunistes (GHESKIO), Port-au-Prince, Haiti

social rejection and are likely to access healthcare or social services late in their disease course if at all (9, 10).

Despite the clear need for targeted and adapted interventions, HIV services for MSM remain severely under-resourced, leading to poor program coverage in many Caribbean countries. This paper aims to present: 1) the HIV infection among MSM in terms of epidemiology, social and cultural factors driving the epidemic, and regional and national responses, and 2) what remains to be addressed to close the gaps in order to identify areas for further research and programme development towards ending AIDS by 2030.

METHODS

To identify peer-reviewed articles, abstracts and reports of HIV studies conducted among MSM in the Caribbean we performed a search of PubMed and Scopus on June 2019 using Medical Subject Headings (MeSH) terms or other associated terms for HIV cross referenced with "stigma", "discrimination reduction", "social stigma", or "homophobia", as well as "men who have sex with men", "gay men", "gay man", "bisexual men", "bisexual man", "homosexual men", "homosexual man", or "homosexuality, male", "high-risk groups", "prevalence", "Caribbean", and individual country names. We considered original research articles, reviews and reports published in English, French and Spanish over the period of January 2009 through May 2019. The 2009-2019 period was selected since an emergence of international interest in the role of MSM in HIV epidemics globally has become more apparent and major innovations took place in HIV testing, prevention, treatment, retention strategies, monitoring and evaluation tools and elimination initiatives.

The initial screening search was based on the titles and abstracts of the articles. Following the search, we reviewed bibliographies of major articles for further references not indexed in the search engine. We also reviewed relevant documents from international organizations such as UNAIDS, Pan Caribbean Partnership against HIV/AIDS (PANCAP) and AIDS case reporting to the Pan American Health Organization (PAHO)/WHO, studies and reports on the social and cultural aspects of Caribbean homosexuality.

For peer-reviewed articles, inclusion criteria were determined a priori: studies including HIV prevalence data, sociocultural risk factors driving the epidemic among MSM; description of regional and national efforts and potential challenges and barriers to effective control of the epidemic among MSM; country report or an abstract at a conference with peer-reviewed blinded abstract selection process; studies from Caribbean region. This report concentrates exclusively on publications related to MSM living in the Caribbean countries.

Each article reviewed was analysed with a standardised tool seeking to identify data on the HIV epidemic among MSM, social and cultural factors, the regional and national responses, the challenges and barriers that remain in the Caribbean. Data were extracted using forms detailing study location, study objectives; thematic areas mentioned above; data collection; methodology (design, setting, population, MSM sample size); results and outcomes; and specific sexual and HIV stigma-related issues. After data extraction for each paper, the studies were grouped and combined with other relevant documents

mentioned above according to the objectives of this review. Narrative summaries are presented below.

RESULTS

The initial search generated 1 644 published articles on HIV in MSM globally. Of that total, 11 peer-reviewed studies, 9 grey literature reports and programme frameworks that specifically referenced HIV in MSM population in the Caribbean and other literatures reporting on homosexuality in the Caribbean were analysed in depth.

The epidemiology of HIV among MSM in the Caribbean

The Caribbean has a global HIV prevalence at 1.2%. Although the HIV transmission is mainly heterosexual it has a concentrated epidemic among key populations such as MSM and sex workers, and MSM accounted for nearly a quarter of new infections in 2017 (5).

High-quality data on HIV prevalence among MSM in the Caribbean is highly limited. Many studies used convenience sampling with very small samples and most provided limited information about the methodologies employed or samples included. Nevertheless, these studies represent an important step forward in countries that obviously had no previous data about HIV prevalence among MSM (11). Although reliability and significant variations in new infections among the countries in the Caribbean region represent a major concern, the prevalence of HIV among MSM is high and the rates also do vary among Caribbean countries. The prevalence is particularly high in Trinidad and Tobago (32.0 %), Bahamas (25.0 %) and Haiti (13.0 %). The lowest prevalence percentages are still high at 5.0 % in Guyana and around 6.0 % in Suriname and Cuba (12).

In 2014, only 51.0 % of MSM were reported to have access to HIV services, a level that has remained unchanged for several years (13). Moreover, access to HIV testing in MSM varies enormously from country to country, ranging from 5.0 % to 70.0 %, and 64.0 % of MSM in Jamaica reported having sexual relationship with women, which also contributed to the spread of HIV in the general population (14, 15).

In recent reports, estimation of the population size of MSM by country, the prevention programmes and antiretroviral treatment coverage among them represented a major challenge (16). Knowledge of HIV status varies between 23.7% in Grenada to 97.5% in Suriname (5), and regular condom use between 42.0 % in the Dominican Republic to 82.0 % in Saint Kitts and Nevis.

Factors underlying the Caribbean HIV epidemic among MSM

Several factors influence the epidemic among MSM in the Caribbean but stigma and discrimination underlie the social vulnerability in driving the HIV epidemic and play a central role. Thus, it is mandatory to catch the social construction of heteronormativity in the region that is also central to the problem because any other form of sexual orientation outside the norm is seen as a deviant act. Therefore, this situation reinforces rejection, ostracism and discrimination.

Homophobia and stigma toward MSM are among the key factors that may be understood in the context of what is socially acceptable to be a man in the Caribbean region. The "heteropatriarchy concept" defines the existing social and political organization in different Caribbean countries, shaped by a history of slavery, colonialism, and a post emancipation nationalism. Heteronormativity can be defined as the institutions, structures, practices, identities, and understanding that legitimize and hierarchize heterosexuality as the normal, natural, and only socially and morally accepted form of sexuality. Thus, an heteronormative and hegemonic model of masculinity is essential to the socialization process and the cultural identity of many Caribbean countries (17).

Caribbean cultural constructions of masculinity impose obligations and restrictions leading to risky sexual practices besides the practice of sex between men remains a criminal offence in most Caribbean countries (18). Highly stigmatized by both religious and social norms, homosexual practices are driven underground. Some men are involved with both male and female sexual partners, and sometimes they appear to adopt a socially acceptable heterosexual lifestyle. Marrying women and fathering children are, for some, a strategy to avoid negative consequences of public disclosure of homosexuality and can be used to help dispel doubts about masculinity. By having female sexual partners, MSM fulfil the traditional gender roles and respect the heteronormative and hegemonic model of masculinity (18). In this way, structural factors are interconnected and converge to increased individual risk practices, thus increasing both social and other individual drivers of HIV vulnerability.

Another factor is violence towards MSM which is not only perpetuated at a community level but also overlooked by police forces. The lack of legal protections contributes to insecurity, including poverty and homelessness for those who are rejected, which elevates HIV vulnerability and decreases access to sexual and HIV information, testing, prevention and care (19).

Moreover, access to prevention, counselling and testing, care and treatment remain difficult in most Caribbean societies (20). Fear of non-voluntary disclosure, confidentiality and a lack of privacy aggravate lack of access (21). Health care providers are perceived as judgmental and unable to respect confidentiality (22). In a study conducted in Jamaica, participants revealed social-ecological barriers to HIV testing. Barriers included healthcare provider mistreatment, confidentiality breaches, and HIV-related stigma. Healthcare provider discrimination and judgment in HIV testing provision presented barriers to accessing HIV services, and resulted in participants hiding their sexual orientation and/or gender identity (23).

Confidentiality concerns included clinical settings that segregated HIV services from other health services, fear that healthcare providers would publicly disclose their status, and concerns at LGBT-friendly clinics that peers would discover they intention to get tested or their HIV status (21). HIV-related stigma contributed to fear of testing HIV-positive; this intersected with the stigma of HIV as a "gay" disease (24). Reports about the difficulties of starting HIV prevention program among MSM in some countries, in correlation with a strong sexual discrimination, lead to legal invisibility of MSM serologic status.

Moreover, studies describe stigmatizing attitudes by university students and health/social service providers towards PLWHIV and LGBT persons in many Caribbean countries, with the highest levels of stigma directed towards MSM living with HIV (24). In another study comparing attitudes of the populations towards MSM in Trinidad and Tobago, Grenada, Guyana, Belize, St. Lucia, Suriname and St Vincent, the attitudes revealed strong homophobic feelings, stigma and discrimination. This also negatively affects the involvement of MSM in successful national HIV responses (25).

Regional and national responses

Even in this non-favourable environment, several international funding programmes such as The President's Emergency Plan for AIDS Relief (PEPFAR), the Global Fund to fight AIDS and the USAID have economically supported the Caribbean countries and have also launched specific initiatives, in partnership with national institutions, to expand MSM's access to and retention in HIV services. In efforts to reach the ambitious 95-95-95 goals of the Joint United Nations Program on HIV/AIDS (UNAIDS) by 2030, MSM are a high priority (26). A strong presence of civil society organisations and community-led networks is also noticed in the Caribbean, with civil society instrumental in both the region's HIV response and human rights activism.

To control the HIV epidemic in the Caribbean MSM patients and those at risk need to flow efficiently, consistently, and sustainably through the entire HIV continuum of prevention, care, and treatment services (27). This seamless integration of interventions requires strong linkages among program components so that HIV transmission is reduced and people diagnosed with HIV obtain early access to antiretroviral treatment and other social supports (27). The Pan American Health Organization (PAHO) has also advocated for combination prevention programs as rights-, evidence-, and community-based programs that promote a combination of biomedical, behavioural, and structural interventions designed to meet the HIV prevention needs of specific people and communities (28).

In terms of HIV testing and prevention, different strategies to testing are being considered and experienced in the region to increase the number of MSM who are aware of their HIV status, but efforts are constrained by health system and policies insufficiently tailored to their needs, health providers layered stigma and limited community-based services (29). HIV self-tests are available in some countries like the Bahamas and Trinidad and Tobago. However, as of 2017, most governments were yet to document their use. This method intends to expand testing to people from key populations like MSM, whose need is significantly greater due to the concentrated nature of the epidemic (28). The regional median for condom use among MSM in their most recent sexual encounter is 63%. All countries provide free condoms to MSM but levels are often inadequate and stigma impedes the distribution flow. Only one third procure condoms using domestic resources. It is essential to increase the availability, access, affordability and use of condoms and also compatible lubricants through targeted distribution schemes (28).

One major recommendation by the World Health Organization (WHO), prior to the start of the International AIDS conference in Melbourne since 2014 was the use of pre-exposure prophylaxis (PrEP) for all MSM as an additional HIV prevention method (30). In 2018, only the Bahamas and Barbados were providing PrEP through the public health system. Although PrEP is available through private providers in the

Dominican Republic, Jamaica and Suriname it is not fully distributed. Efforts are also noted in Cuba, Dominica and Haiti so it can be fully implemented (31).

Persistent challenges

The conservative nature of Caribbean societies makes it difficult to identify, define and reach MSM groups. This is compounded by the limited availability of disaggregated data, particularly in smaller countries where health information and monitoring systems are not well developed or controlled rigorously. Many countries report data on MSM, and despite high rates of population mobility in the region, there is very little data on HIV prevalence among migrant and mobile populations. Further, the vast majority of countries do not collect or report data for subgroups of stigmatised and isolated populations who often face multiple and overlapping vulnerabilities and risks. These include non-identifying MSM and MSM sex workers who do and do not identify as homosexual (32).

Barriers to testing for MSM are still numerous. For example, in the majority of the countries, testing centres are concentrated in large cities or in localities where confidentiality seems to be an issue. Besides, almost all the countries provide sensitivity training for health workers involved in HIV screening and care for MSM, but civil society organisations that participated in national consultations on HIV prevention reported a lack of sensitivity among these professionals besides the absence of LGBT issues in medical curriculum (28).

PANCAP has led and coordinated advocacy efforts to accelerate the human rights agenda and to eliminate stigma and discrimination. Although all Caribbean states have integrated some elements of human rights in their national response to HIV, in many instances new policies are not being fully implemented. In spite of these efforts, stigma and discrimination persist. Recent surveys of health facilities on three islands have found stigma and discriminatory practices present across all levels of staff (33).

Although progresses have been reported, the Anglophone Caribbean has maintained some of the most regressive anti-homosexual laws in the world. Same-gender intimacy, regardless of consent or physical location, was criminalised in 11 Caribbean Community (CARICOM) states. Sentences ranged from life imprisonment in Barbados and Guyana to 10 years in Belize, Dominica, Grenada, St. Kitts and Nevis, and St Vincent and the Grenadines. There were also laws against cross-dressing and constitutional bans on legal recognition of same-sex relationships. Trinidad and Tobago prohibited entry for homosexuals (34).

Weaknesses in health systems continue to present barriers to access and sustainability of services, particularly where parallel service delivery systems for HIV have been established. Vertical systems are inefficient, costly and perpetuate stigma and discrimination, resulting in low rates of entry and retention in treatment. Of major concern is the loss of patients at various stages along the HIV treatment continuum, as this reduces the proportion achieving viral suppression (28).

Intra-Caribbean migration, including high levels of transnational mobility and return migration, may increase the vulnerability of certain migrant subpopulations including MSM who face a range of barriers to accessing health services (33).

Many countries continue to face deficiencies in research capacity and in translating findings into actionable recommendations for policy and programme development (35).

Finally, the Caribbean region is characterised by a wide range of economic and human development levels which can have a huge impact on HIV care for the general population, including MSM. While some Caribbean states have developed-country status, at the other end of the spectrum we find some with low-income status. In between these extremes, many countries are all classified as middle-income, in spite of their vastly different economies and high levels of vulnerability to external shocks. Vulnerability resulting from the lack of economic diversity and heavy reliance on international funders and donors for HIV programmes is compounded by limited in-country institutional capacities (32).

DISCUSSION

Although homosexuality is not viewed the same in all the Caribbean countries, it is largely related to a person´s beliefs about its origins. According to a study conducted in Barbados, Guyana and Trinidad and Tobago, attitudes towards homosexuality are grounded in strong rooted stereotypes. Therefore, although there is tolerance in certain social classes, MSM are often perceived as sources of both symbolic and realistic threat to society.

This report showed that MSM face a disproportionate share of the HIV epidemic in the Caribbean region relative to the general population. In many countries, the HIV risk to MSM is exacerbated by social, cultural, and political factors. These include cultural biases against MSM; limited access to information and services; low national investments in health; and legal, institutional or social barriers, including negative bias among providers, that make it difficult for MSM to negotiate safe sex or obtain adequate healthcare services. This situation is also compounded by adverse human rights environments that still prevail in many countries in the Caribbean where MSM may fail to seek treatment.

Among MSM, HIV rates are unacceptably high and could provide a reservoir for further and increased HIV spread among Caribbean general population. Nevertheless, these data must be interpreted with caution due to significant under-reporting from many countries as well as a considerable lag in reporting from some countries. Special measures need to be taken by health authorities and regional organisations to build bridges with the MSM community and empower them to promote safe sex and reduce HIV infection rates.

Reducing the high HIV prevalence among MSM in the Caribbean remains one of the most critical challenges in effectively controlling the HIV epidemic. It is unlikely that this will be feasible with current methods of prevention and treatment unless significant progress is made in reducing the strong stigma associated with homosexuality, removing the structural barriers to them accessing social services, addressing their social vulnerability, and empowering them to practice safe sex. A clear response to improve the legal/human rights environment affecting sexual diversity is needed in the Caribbean, not only on grounds of progress of the international agenda on human rights, but also based on a public health and development perspective. Multisectoral efforts should be made to show the social harm of homophobic laws and practices, and to generate initiatives leading to positive changes (32, 33, 35).

In the Caribbean, renewed commitment to combination prevention and treatment that is tailored to MSM is urgently needed to be fully implemented and closely monitored to accelerate reductions in new HIV infections by strong prevention programmes and increase retention in care for those on antiretroviral treatment.

Another important point is achieving the funding required to end the AIDS epidemic. This will demand renewed international commitment, innovative financing and an intensified strategic focus. Low-income Caribbean countries, especially those with a heavy HIV burden, will need substantial international support to ensure rapid scale-up to end the epidemic.

Conclusions

The prevalence of HIV among MSM is high and the rates also do vary among Caribbean countries. Several factors influence the epidemic among MSM in the Caribbean but stigma and discrimination underlie the social vulnerability in driving the HIV epidemic and play a central role. To end the AIDS epidemic by 2030, the global community will need to defy expectations in terms of tolerance and solidarity. MSM can no longer be kept unchecked in the era of the Sustainable Development Goals with the motto 'Leave no one behind' while working towards a world free of HIV.

Authors' contributions. WD and YC conceived the original research idea and led the design of the study. All authors developed the protocol. WD and YC conducted the analysis. WD developed the first draft of the article. All authors oversaw the development of the article and contributed to the revisions. All authors reviewed and approved the final draft.

Conflicts of interest. None declared.

Disclaimer. Authors hold sole responsibility for the views expressed in the manuscript, which may not necessarily reflect the opinion or policy of the *RPSP/PAJPH* and/or PAHO.

REFERENCES

1. Global AIDS Monitoring 2019 [Internet]. United Nations Digital Library System. 2020 [cited 7 July 2020]. Available from: https://digitallibrary.un.org/record/3801751
2. The Joint United Nations Programme on HIV/AIDS (UNAIDS) Data 2019 [Internet]. Public Health Update. 2020 [cited 7 July 2020]. Available from: https://www.publichealthupdate.com/the-joint-united-nations-programme-on-hiv-aids-unaids-data-2019/
3. Linger D. Bodies, Pleasures, and Passions: Sexual Culture in Contemporary Brazil. RICHARD G. PARKER. American Ethnologist. 1994;21(4):1092-1093.
4. Caceres C, Rosasco A. The margin has many sides: Diversity among gay and homosexually active men in Lima. Culture, Health & Sexuality. 1999;1(3):261-275.
5. Beyrer C, Baral S, van Griensven F, Goodreau S, Chariyalertsak S, Wirtz A et al. Global epidemiology of HIV infection in men who have sex with men. Lancet. 2012;380(9839):367-77.
6. Senior K. HIV, human rights, and men who have sex with men. Lancet Infect Dis. 2010;10(7):448-449.
7. Jackman M. They called it the 'abominable crime': an analysis of heterosexual support for anti-gay laws in Barbados, Guyana and Trinidad and Tobago. Sex Res Soc Policy. 2015;13(2):130-141.
8. Ayala G, Makofane K, Santos G, Beck J, Do T, Hebert P et al. Access to Basic HIV-Related Services and PrEP Acceptability among Men Who Have sex with Men Worldwide: Barriers, Facilitators, and Implications for Combination Prevention. J Sex Transm Dis. 2013;2013:1-11.
9. AIDSinfo | UNAIDS [Internet]. Aidsinfo.unaids.org. 2020 [cited 28 September 2020]. Available from: http://aidsinfo.unaids.org/
10. Figueroa J. Review of HIV in the Caribbean: Significant Progress and Outstanding Challenges. Current HIV/AIDS Reports. 2014;11(2):158-167.
11. Maiorana A, Rebchook G, Kassie N, Myers J. On Being Gay in Barbados: "Bullers" and "Battyboys" and their HIV Risk in a Societal Context of Stigma. J Homosex. 2013;60(7):984-1010.
12. UNAIDS [Internet]. Unaids.org. 2020 [cited 28 September 2020]. Available from: http://www.unaids.org/en/resources/documents/2017/2017_data_book.
13. Logie C, Wang Y, Marcus N, Levermore K, Jones N, Ellis T et al. Pathways From Sexual Stigma to Inconsistent Condom Use and Condom Breakage and Slippage Among MSM in Jamaica. J Acquir Immune Defic Syndr. 2018;78(5):513-521.
14. Britton C. Review: Opacity: Gender, Sexuality, Race, and the 'Problem' of Identity in Martinique. French Studies. 2003;57(3):426-427.
15. De Boni R, Veloso V, Grinsztejn B. Epidemiology of HIV in Latin America and the Caribbean. Curr Opin HIV AIDS. 2014;9(2):192-198.
16. Masculine Norms and Violence: Making the Connections | Promundo [Internet]. Promundo. 2020 [cited 28 September 2020]. Available from: https://promundoglobal.org/resources/masculine-norms-violence-making-connections/
17. Figueroa J. High HIV Prevalence among Men Who Have Sex with Men in Jamaica is Associated with Social Vulnerability and Other Sexually Transmitted Infections. West Indian Med J. 2013;62(4):286-91.
18. Rodríguez-Díaz CE, Jovet-Toledo GG, Vélez-Vega CM, et al. Discrimination and Health among Lesbian, Gay, Bisexual and Trans People in Puerto Rico. P R Health Sci J. 2016 Sep;35(3):154-9.
19. Beck EJ, Mandalia S, Barrow C, Massiah E, Nunez C. Attitudes towards Key Populations in Three Fast Track Caribbean Countries: Haiti, Jamaica and the Dominican Republic. J HIV AIDS. 2018;4(3).
20. Rogers S, Tureski K, Cushnie A, Brown A, Bailey A, Palmer Q. Layered stigma among health-care and social service providers toward key affected populations in Jamaica and The Bahamas. AIDS Care. 2013;26(5):538-546.
21. Logie C, Lacombe-Duncan A, Brien N, Jones N, Lee-Foon N, Levermore K et al. Barriers and facilitators to HIV testing among young men who have sex with men and transgender women in Kingston, Jamaica: a qualitative study. J Int AIDS Soc. 2017;20(1):21385.
22. Abell N, Rutledge S, McCann T, Padmore J. Examining HIV/AIDS provider stigma: assessing regional concerns in the islands of the Eastern Caribbean. AIDS Care. 2007;19(2):242-247.
23. Beck E, Espinosa K, Ash T, Wickham P, Barrow C, Massiah E et al. Attitudes towards homosexuals in seven Caribbean countries: implications for an effective HIV response. AIDS Care. 2017;29(12):1557-1566.
24. Rutledge S, Abell N, Padmore J, McCann T. AIDS stigma in health services in the Eastern Caribbean. Sociol Health Illn. 2009;31(1):17-34.
25. Francis C, Mills S. HIV Cascade Framework for Key Populations. 2015. [cited 28 September 2020]. Available from: https://www.fhi360.org/sites/default/files/media/documents/linkages-hiv-cascade-framework-oct15.pdf
26. HIV Prevention in the Spotlight [Internet]. Paho.org. 2020 [cited 28 September 2020]. Available from: https://www.paho.org/hiv-prevention-spotlight-2017/
27. Rodríguez MM, Madera SR, Díaz NV. Stigma and Homophobia: Persistent Challenges for HIV Prevention Among Young MSM in Puerto Rico. Rev Cienc Soc. 2013;26:50-59
28. PAHO/WHO. HIV Prevention and Comprehensive Care for Key Populations - Scientific and Technical Materials [Internet]. Washington, DC: PAHO/WHO; 2020 [cited 28 September 2020]. Available from: https://www.paho.org/hq/index.php?option=

com_content&view=article&id=13964:hiv-prevention-comprehen-sive-care-key-populations-documents&Itemid=72171&lang=en

29. DeVita T, Bishop C, Plankey M. Queering medical education: systematically assessing LGBTQI health competency and implementing reform. Med Educ Online. 2018;23(1):1510703.

30. Dudar K, Ghaderi G, Gallant J, Dickinson J, Abourbih J, Briggs M. Queering the Medical Curriculum: How to Design, Develop, Deliver and Assess Learning Outcomes Relevant to LGBT Health for Health Care Professionals. MedEdPublish. 2018;7(1).

31. Prevent HIV, test and treat all - WHO support for country impact [Internet]. World Health Organization. 2020 [cited 28 September 2020]. Available from: https://www.who.int/hiv/pub/progressreports/2016-progress-report/en/

32. Stigma Reduction Framework for HIV and AIDS : National Actions to Reduce HIV-Related Stigma & Discrimination and Improve Health Outcomes Understanding Stigma and Discrimination [Internet]. Healthpolicyproject.com. 2020 [cited 28 September 2020]. Available from: https://www.healthpolicyproject.com/pubs/143_PANCAPStigmaFramework.pdf

33. Rouzier V, Farmer P, Pape J, Jerome J, Van Onacker J, Morose W et al. Factors impacting the provision of antiretroviral therapy to people living with HIV: the view from Haiti. Antiviral Therapy. 2014;19(Suppl 3):91-104.

34. Beyrer C. Strategies to manage the HIV epidemic in gay, bisexual, and other men who have sex with men. Curr Opin Infect Dis. 2014;27(1):1-8.

35. Cáceres C. HIV among gay and other men who have sex with men in Latin America and the Caribbean: a hidden epidemic? AIDS. 2002;16:S23-S33.

Manuscript received on 4 March 2020. Revised version accepted for publication on 6 November 2020.

La infección por el VIH en hombres que tienen relaciones sexuales con hombres en el Caribe: alcanzar a los que quedaron atrás

RESUMEN

Objetivos. Presentar los factores epidemiológicos, sociales y culturales que impulsan la epidemia de la infección por el VIH en los hombres que tienen relaciones sexuales con hombres (HSH) en el Caribe, así como destacar las respuestas a nivel nacional y regional y las brechas que deben cerrarse para poner fin a la epidemia de sida para el 2030.

Métodos. Se realizó una revisión bibliográfica a partir de búsquedas en las siguientes bases de datos: PubMed y Scopus. Se seleccionaron artículos publicados en los últimos diez años que abordan los factores de riesgo socioculturales, la descripción de las iniciativas nacionales y regionales, y los posibles retos y obstáculos al control eficaz de la epidemia en los HSH. Este informe se centra exclusivamente en aquellas publicaciones sobre los HSH en los países del Caribe.

Resultados. Se realizó un análisis temático de 11 estudios arbitrados y 9 artículos y marcos programáticos de la bibliografía gris. La prevalencia de la infección por el VIH en los HSH es alta y las tasas varían entre los países del Caribe. Existen varios factores que influyen en la epidemia de la infección por el VIH en los HSH en el Caribe, pero el estigma y la discriminación están en el centro de la vulnerabilidad social y ayudan a impulsar la epidemia.

Conclusiones. En la era de los Objetivos de Desarrollo Sostenible y su lema de "no dejar a nadie atrás", no se puede continuar desatendiendo a los HSH si se quiere poner fin a la epidemia de sida para el 2030.

Palabras clave   VIH; enfermedades de transmisión sexual; equidad; Región del Caribe.

HIV em homens que fazem sexo com homens no Caribe: alcançando os que ficaram para trás

RESUMO

Objetivos. Descrever o perfil epidemiológico e fatores socioculturais determinantes da epidemia de HIV em homens que fazem sexo com homens (HSH) na região do Caribe e chamar atenção para as respostas nacionais e regionais e o que ainda falta para suprir as falhas e eliminar a aids até 2030.

Métodos. Uma revisão da literatura foi realizada nas bases de dados PubMed e Scopus com a seleção de artigos publicados nos 10 últimos anos. Os desfechos de interesse foram fatores de risco socioculturais, descrição das iniciativas nacionais e regionais e potenciais desafios e obstáculos ao controle efetivo da epidemia de HIV em HSH. O estudo se restringiu exclusivamente a publicações relativas a HSH vivendo nos países do Caribe.

Resultados. Onze estudos avaliados por pares e 9 relatos da literatura cinzenta e enquadramentos de programas foram analisados tematicamente. A prevalência do HIV é alta em HSH vivendo no Caribe e os índices variam entre os países. Diversos fatores influenciam a epidemia em HSH, mas o estigma e a discriminação constituem a base da vulnerabilidade social e têm um papel central na epidemia do HIV no Caribe.

Conclusões. Para eliminar a epidemia de aids até 2030, os HSH não podem mais ficar sem monitoração na era dos Objetivos de Desenvolvimento Sustentável com sua missão de "não deixar ninguém para trás".

Palavras-chave   HIV; doenças sexualmente transmissíveis; equidade; Região do Caribe.

Presentation of the study 2:

The prior study aimed to present: 1) the HIV infection among MSM in terms of epidemiology, social and cultural factors driving the epidemic, and regional and national responses, and 2) what remains to be addressed to close the gaps in order to identify areas for further research and programme development towards ending AIDS by 2030. While it allowed us to capture the context in which MSM are living in the Caribbean, it also presented the major program framework strategies and interventions with respect to the macro, meso and micro levels. We explored the environmental and social influences in the Caribbean, the country-specific situation and the national/regional response.

After this scoping description, it is essential to bring the exploration at the health system's level by exploring the impact of stigma on the continuum of HIV services. Therefore, the study 2 will aimed to analyze scientific publications to assess what is known about stigma and discrimination from the perspective of MSM living with, what is the impact on the continuum of care and what interventions and/or programs have been developed to address stigma.

Study 2:

Impact of Stigma on the continuum of HIV services for Men who have Sex with Men in the Caribbean and Africa

3.1.2.1

Introduction

HIV related stigma to Men who have Sex with Men (MSM) in the Caribbean and Africa, the two most affected regions in the world, remain a major barrier for effective prevention and treatment programs. Stigma description, measurement, and reduction interventions are crucial to the HIV success response. This paper aimed to review the scientific literature on MSM living with HIV related stigma to document the current state of research.

Methods

Following specific inclusion criteria this review included studies related to the description of stigma and intervention efforts developed in the Caribbean and Africa and indexed in the PubMed database from march 2008 to march 2018.

Results

Of 1179 articles identified, 40 studies were included in our review. The studies targeted MSM, Health-care-workers (HCW), health students and the general population in 29 countries of which 33 (82,5%) conducted in Africa and 7 (17,5%) in the Caribbean. The description studies showed relationship between stigma and HIV risk factors, prevention, treatment, socialization and human rights. The interventions targeted MSM and HCW with community actions and training strategies. Although stigma measurement tools lacked uniformity and validity the majority of intervention studies were effective at reducing the aspects of stigma they treated.

Conclusion

Our review gave a large volume of information and comprehensiveness related to HIV infected MSM related stigma description and interventions. Considering the negative impact of stigma on MSM health, it is an evidence that stakeholders need to completely address this issue in order to control the HIV epidemic.

Keywords: literature review; MSM; HIV; stigma; discrimination; description; interventions; measurement.

3.1.2.2 Introduction

Since the beginning of the epidemic, HIV is a disease that has been associated with social stigma (1). Stigma against people living with HIV, especially sexual minorities, reinforces marginalization and makes access to care difficult (2). According to Canadian sociologist Ervin Goffman (1963), one of the earliest scholars to theorize stigma, it is any personal attribute, real or perceived, that conveys a negative social identity, thus devaluing the person's social position. The Joint United Nations Program on HIV/AIDS describes stigma as "a process of devaluation of people either living with, or associated with, HIV and AIDS" (3). This condition is considered a major barrier to effective responses to the HIV epidemic (4). Despite public education programs and equal rights legislation, stigmatization continues to be widespread and can affect many aspects of life (5).

Men who have sex with men (MSM) are among the community populations throughout the world that have been one of the constituencies most affected by HIV, and continue to be one of the population groups most vulnerable to infection and death related to HIV because they engage in high-risk sexual behaviour (6–8). MSM living with HIV are subjected to a plethora of unpleasant treatment that includes discrimination, social ostracism and violence (9). As a result, the social, emotional and relational aspects of their lives are sometimes extremely affected, leading to marginalization (2). In addition to this, stigmatization as gay and fear of being HIV-positive present barriers to making use of the available voluntary HIV testing and counselling services (10). Experienced stigma is the actual experience or occurrence of discrimination, such as denial of health care services or the criminalization of same-sex practices. These forms of stigma play a role in the lives of MSM and within the context of the HIV epidemic (11).

MSM are inadequately studied in many countries, and despite well-characterized risks for HIV acquisition and transmission, they continue to be under-represented in national HIV surveillance systems, in targeted prevention programs, and in care (12). The global response to the pandemic has progressed over the decades both in scale and in efforts to reach diverse and vulnerable groups, stigma and discrimination still follow MSM in many settings (13). While much of the literature has focused on identifying factors that affect HIV rates among MSM, a few tried to identify interventions that consider the MSM specificities regarding social contexts and cultures (14).

Stigma: Definition and Conceptualization

As a process of devaluation that exclude, reject, blame or devalue individuals in the eyes of others, the definition of "stigma" is variable in the literature (15,16) (16). This dynamic concept is approached from different theoretical views that led to different conceptualizations (17). Link defined stigma as a social process that exists when elements of labelling, stereotyping, separation, status loss, and discrimination occur in a power situation that allows them (17). Weiss and Ramakrishna went further by describing it as a related personal experience characterized by exclusion, rejection, blame or devaluation that   results from experience or reasonable anticipation of an adverse social judgement about a person or group. In health-related stigma, this judgment is based on an enduring feature of identity conferred by a health problem or health related condition (18).

Goffman distinguished three types of stigma: physical deformity, character blemishes and prejudice. The second one may occur in individuals with HIV/AIDS. For example, individuals infected with HIV/AIDS face considerable stigma because many believe that the infected person could have controlled the behaviors that resulted in the infection (19). In addition to this, some groups, identities, and behaviours are consistently stigmatized across much of the world. Examples include stigma based on: sexual practices and identities of gay men and other men who have sex with men (MSM) (20). In many cases, for men who have sex with men, HIV/AIDS poses a double burden—on the one hand, there are a very limited number of programmes specifically designed to reach them, and on the other hand, they are often faced with discrimination, stigma and in some cases even criminal prosecution by the societies they live in (21). Stigma is, thus, enacted and perceived through social processes, violence, aggression and family rejection (22).

In this paper, we aimed to review the published literature to examine what is known about stigma and discrimination of HIV-infected MSM, what is the impact of these issues on the continuum of care and what interventions and/or programs have been developed to address them in two regions in the world: Africa and the Caribbean. These two regions were chosen based on the fact they are the most HIV affected area and they share some similarities in terms of ethnography.

The following questions informed the review guideline: How stigma and discrimination affect the continuum of care of HIV-positive MSM in Africa and the Caribbean? What interventions have been doing so far? While studying the impact, we also critically examined the literature to elucidate the relationship of stigma to the successfulness of HIV prevention and treatment programs. Finally, we synthesized the interventions.

3.1.2.3 Methods

Research questions and objectives

In line with the research questions, articles that correlated Stigma, MSM and HIV were identified. The collection period occurred in March and April 2018. Articles published between march 2008 and march 2018 were surveyed. The analysis followed the predetermined eligibility criteria.

Search strategy and articles selection

In march 2018, PubMed search for all published articles pertaining to HIV/AIDS infected MSM related stigma was run. To perform as broad a search as possible, the search term "(stigma*[Title/abstract] OR discrimination*[Title/abstract] OR "Discrimination (Psychology)"[MeSH Terms] OR "Social Stigma"[MeSH Terms] OR "Prejudice"[MeSH Terms]) AND (HIV[Title/abstract] OR seropositive[Title/abstract] OR AIDS[Title/abstract] OR "HIV Infections"[MeSH Terms]) AND ("men who have sex with men"[Title/abstract] OR "gay men"[Title/abstract] OR "gay man"[Title/abstract] OR "bisexual men"[Title/abstract] OR "bisexual man"[Title/abstract] OR "homosexual men"[Title/abstract] OR "homosexual man"[Title/abstract] OR "Homosexuality, Male"[MeSH Terms])" was utilized. Then the 10-year period and the human species filters were applied. This timeframe of a decade was used to provide sufficient historical perspective on trends in stigma measurement and developed interventions. Each of the abstracts identified was reviewed. Following the PubMed search, bibliographies of major articles for further references not indexed in the search engine were reviewed.

The following four criteria had to be met in order to include a study in this review: the study is conducted in Africa or the Caribbean; the study subjects include MSM and include results separately about MSM (either attitudes, behaviors, outcomes about MSM or from MSM); Stigma or discrimination is reported as an exposure or outcome, its relationship to people with HIV or MSM is addressed in the study; the study is about HIV, either its prevention or treatment, access to care, affordability of care, or health care structures related to HIV infected patients. We also included studies that lacked a clear description of the measures used or those that used non-validated measures for stigma.

Screening and data abstraction

Article citations were organized, uploaded and reviewed using excel spreadsheet. The title, author, journal and year of publication were then exported for title and abstract review. Abstracts were screened to determine whether they included relevant information. If the abstract was deemed compatible, the full article was then retrieved and screened for relevant information. If the full text had to be obtained to determine if the abstract was relevant, the full text was reviewed.

From each article, data were obtained on: the design of the study, either it was quantitative, qualitative or mixed-method; date of data collection; country of the study; location where data were collected (healthcare setting or community); the main objective; the targets ; the sample size; the type of stigma measured, analysed or mentioned (perceived, enacted or both); the stigma scale used if stigma was measured; the study purpose (description or intervention); the outcomes and the main findings. If any of the data mentioned could not be obtained or was not mentioned, we then classified it as "not specified".

3.1.2.4 Results

The search criteria identified 1179 potentially relevant articles. After removing 410 from the human subject, 10-years period, African and Caribbean location filters, 147 abstracts were retained for review. After the review, a total of 40 articles met the inclusion criteria and were included for data abstraction.

The flowchart of screening process for inclusion of articles describing stigma and/or interventions for better health outcome of HIV-infected men who have sex with men (MSM) in the Caribbean and Africa is well described in table 1.

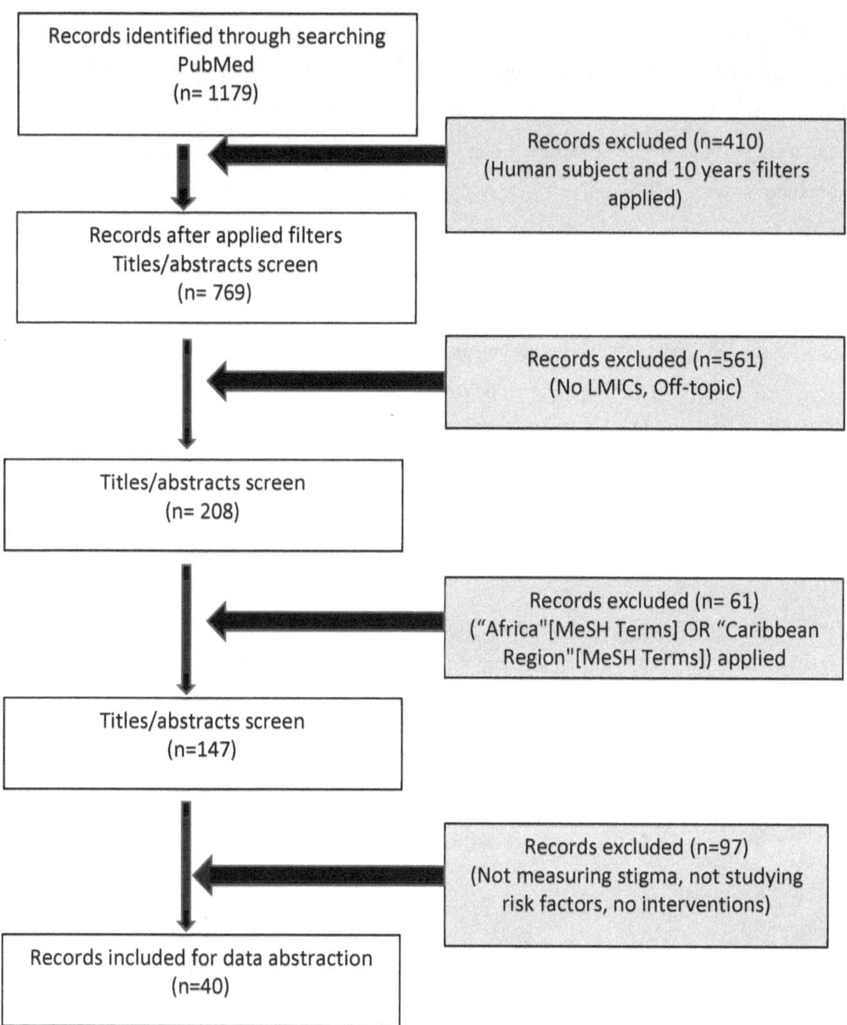

Figure 1. Flowchart of the articles' selection

LMICs: Low and Middle-Income Countries

Characteristics of the study

Region: In terms of localization, the studies spanned from Africa and the Caribbean with most of them in Africa 33 (82,5%), and 7 (17,5%) from the Caribbean. Among the African one, most of the studies came from western and eastern Africa, Kenya represents the country with the most followed by Swaziland and South Africa. Most of the Caribbean studies took part in Jamaica. Location: The studies took place mainly in community facilities 30 (75%) and healthcare settings 6 (15%) and only one was done in prison. Target population: The target populations were MSM only in 25 (62%), healthcare workers only in 7 (17%) and a combination of the two in 6 (15%) while only 2 (5%) tried to have a view from MSM from the general population. Purpose: 7 (17,5%) describe and/or tested interventions to reduce stigma and to better engage MSM in care while 33 (82,5%) only describe and/or mentioned stigma as an outcome. 8 (20%) of the studies measured stigma. Both types of stigma (enacted and perceived) were described, mentioned or measured in 30 (75%) of the studies. Methods: The methods used were mainly quantitative 22 (55%). 14 (35 %) used qualitative interviews and focus groups and 3 (7,5%) were mixed-methods studies

Table 1. General characteristics of the studies included		
Characteristics		N (%)
Location	Healthcare settings	6 (15%)
	Community	30 (75%)
	Both	3 (7,5%)
	Others	1 (2,5%)
Target population	MSM only	25 (62%)
	Healthcare workers only	7 (17%)
	Community members	2 (5%)
	MSM + Healthcare workers	6 (15%)
Types of stigma	Enacted	6 (15%)
	Perceived	4 (10%)
	Enacted + Perceived	30 (75%)
Method	Quantitative	22 (55%)
	Qualitative	14 (35 %)
	Mixed Methods	3 (7,5%)
	Intervention description	1 (2,5%)
Study purpose	Description	33 (82,5%)
	Intervention	7 (17,5%)

Stigma measure	Yes	8 (20%)
	No	32 (80%)
Geographic regions	Caribbean	7 (17,5%)
	Africa	33 (82,5%)

Impact of stigma on the continuum

Impact on stigma on HIV risk factors and prevention

Sexual activity is influenced by the strict social taboo against homosexuality and MSM appeared to conceal their sexual relationships. (23). As a consequence, some personal and societal factors put MSM at risk of HIV infection: multiple concurrent partnerships, and short-term relationships, decision on condom use, misconception about anal sex, perceived and experienced stigma at healthcare facilities from healthcare workers and derogatory terms by family, church or community members (24,25). Although they express a need for support from friends, family members and healthcare providers, they are fearful of being stigmatized and rejected if they disclosed their sexual orientation. (25).

HCW response are sometimes barriers to clinic treatment for genital and anal STI that may have implications in HIV infection (26–29). MSM believe that health care providers' lack of understanding of their specific psychosocial issues, vulnerabilities to particular infections, and preventative health needs, limited their ability to provide valuable information to enable them to take control of their own health. Service providers, on the other hand, feel that despite their growing experience, more targeted training would have been helpful to improve their effectiveness in MSM-specific risk reduction counselling (30,31).

Table 2. Summary of stigma, HIV risk factors and prevention studies

1st Author	Country	sample size	Main findings
Logie CH	Jamaica	556 MSM	There's a significantly higher level of perceived and enacted stigma among MSM facing increased social marginalization
Sithole B	Swaziland	50 MSM	A part of self-stigma that put MSM at higher risk of HIV, healthcare facilities'

			heteronormative settings make it difficult for them to disclose.
Poteat T	Burkina Faso, Côte d'Ivoire, Gambia, Lesotho, Malawi, Senegal, Swaziland, Togo	4586 MSM	Gender diversity needs to be addressed within HIV research and programs.
Kushwaha S	Ghana	137 MSM, 32 HCP	MSM are exposed to negative health care climates undermined by a generally unsupportive cultural and social context.
Ruisenor-Escudero H	Togo	354 MSM	Need for evidence-based and human-rights affirming combination HIV prevention and treatment programs that address the various risk levels for MSM
Larsson M	Tanzania	100 MSM	Sexual stigma is a main driver of sexual risk practices among MSM.
Ross MW	Tanzania	200 MSM	Stigma and negative HCW responses are barriers to public clinic treatment for MSM.
Wendi D	Lesotho	318 MSM	Alcohol use and depressive symptoms due to stigma mediate the relationship between MSM stigma in the health care system.
Brown CA	Swaziland	326 MSM	Facing legal discrimination is associated HIV risk factors.
Muzyamba C	Zambia	7 MSM, 10 HCW	Need for human rights programs to address the complex drivers of the HIV epidemic.
Schwartz SR	Nigeria	707 MSM	The negative effects of HIV treatment and care in MSM reinforce the unintended consequences of such legislation on global goals of HIV eradication
Nelson LE	Ghana	137 MSM	Need for the development of intervention programs that address HIV prevention knowledge gaps and reduce HIV stigma against MSM in communities.

Tucker A	South Africa	316 MSM	HIV prevention programs aimed at sexual minority groups should be mindful of potentially complex relationships between social stigmas such as homophobia and sexual risk-taking behaviour.
Taegtmeyer M	Kenya	16 HCW	Service providers felt that despite their growing experience, more targeted training would have been helpful to improve their effectiveness in MSM-specific risk reduction counselling.
Vu L	South Africa	324 MSM	High levels of internalized homophobia exist among South African MSM. A greater level of internalized homophobia was significantly associated with a lower level of education a higher level of HIV misinformation, bisexual identity (vs. homosexual), and HIV-related conspiracy beliefs.
Baral S	Lesotho	252 MSM	HIV knowledge was low; only 3.7% of MSM knew that receptive anal intercourse was the highest risk for HIV and that a water-based lubricant was most appropriate to use with condoms. Human rights abuses were common: 76.2% reported at least one abuse, including rape, blackmail, fear of seeking healthcare, police discrimination, verbal or physical harassment, or having been beaten

Impact of stigma on HIV testing and treatment

Fear of knowing their HIV status and the social consequences thereafter are cited as major deterrents to HIV testing that is also undermined by fatalist views and perceived as a death sentence (32). Experiences of, and fear of, mistreatment by healthcare providers and other medical staff is a barrier to accessing HIV testing where MSM often hide their sexual orientation and/or gender identity (33). Confidentiality is also a concern as some clinics separated patients coming for an HIV test in an area from persons seeking other health services.

(33). HIV-related stigma contributes to fear of testing and receiving a positive result. The stigma of HIV as a "gay disease" and fear of seeking health care services in settings that criminalize same-sex practices also produce a barrier to HIV testing (34).

Wanyenze described nine major barriers to HIV treatment and adherence: "Negative attitudes and unwelcoming behaviors of health workers and the healthcare environment; Health care workers' lack of sufficient skills and knowledge to manage MSM-specific health care needs; Negative community perceptions towards MSM; fear of being segregated or exposed as MSM; limited access to MSM-specific services; high mobility of MSM population, lack of national-level guidelines on how to deal with MSM; a harsh legal environment; and general fears related to HIV-associated stigma and HIV testing" (35). These conditions lead to rejection of conventional care services in favor of faith-healing and herbal medications and nondisclosure which is an important step in the provision of appropriate healthcare (36).

Table 3. Summary of stigma, HIV testing and treatment studies

1st Author	Country	sample size	Main findings
Logie CH	Jamaica	30 MSM, 28 Transgender women	Interventions to challenge stigma in community and healthcare settings can enhance access to the HIV prevention cascade among MSM.
Micheni M	Kenya	29 HCW	HCWs noted challenges specific to MSM: lack of access to MSM-friendly health services, economic and social challenges due to stigma, difficult relationships with care providers, and discrimination at the clinic and in the community.
Shangani S	Kenya	89 MSM	Development of MSM- sensitive HIV testing services, addressing stigma, and training healthcare workers to provide culturally sensitive services may assist in effectively engaging MSM in the HIV treatment cascade.
Wanyenze RK	Uganda	85 MSM, 61 community members	MSM are not comfortable disclosing their sexual orientation to providers and feel providers do not respect them.

Duvall S	Burkina Faso, Togo	38 community members	Several policy barriers restrict MSM from accessing services. Laws criminalizing MSM, particularly anti-solicitation laws, result in harassment and arrests. Public stigma and discrimination create a hostile enabling environment.
Wirtz AL	Malawi	8 MSM, 5 HCW	Results highlight disclosure fears among MSM and, among providers, a lack of awareness and self-efficacy to provide care in the face of limited information and political support.
Rogers SJ	Jamaica, Bahamas	332 HCW	While results across the study's character vignettes generally reflected low levels of stigma, they did demonstrate a pattern of layered stigma. The highest stigma levels were for characters who were MSM as well as living with HIV.
Kennedy CE	Swaziland	46 MSM	Perceived and experienced stigma from healthcare settings, particularly around sexual identity, also led to delayed care-seeking, travel to more distant clinics and missed opportunities for appropriate services.
Risher K	Swaziland	323 MSM	Stigma is common, including fear of seeking healthcare, enacted stigma and perceived social stigma (family, friends). This has an impact on disclosure and engagement to healthcare.
Andrinopoul	Jamaica	25 MSM	Participant narratives unveil a purposeful manipulation of beliefs related to homosexuality that impedes an effective response to HIV and AIDS both in prison and wider society. Findings indicate that homophobia is both a social construction and a tangible tool used to leverage power and a sense of solidarity in a larger political and economic landscape.

Okall DO	Kenya	65 MSM	Over 60% of survey MSM participants were not very comfortable seeking health services from a public hospital. Almost all MSM reported willingness to be contacted to participate in future HIV research studies.

Impact of stigma on socialization, violence and human rights

The homophobic views express by the African and Caribbean cultures result in stigma and discrimination by members of the general public towards MSM. This negatively affects the involvement of MSM in successful national HIV responses (37). Homosexuality is represented as a dangerous threat to the religious, moral, and demographic social order that must be combated (22).

Some countries adopt Same-Sex Marriage Prohibition Act, then gay men and MSM experience increased stigma and discrimination in the period immediately after the signing of this act. (38). MSM have reported multiple forms of abuse perpetrated by police officers (39). Even in the presence of a supportive donor and political community, public stigma and discrimination create a hostile enabling environment (40). Findings indicate that homophobia is both a social construction and a tangible tool used to leverage power and a sense of solidarity in a larger political and economic landscape (41).

Table 4. Summary of stigma, socialization, violence and human rights' studies

1st Author	Country	sample size	Main findings
Beck EJ	St Vincent, Grenada, Guyana, Trinidad, St Lucia, Belize, Suriname	6037 MSM	The homophobic views expressed by these cultures result in stigma and discrimination by members of the "general" public towards MSM negatively affects their involvement in successful national HIV responses
Winskell K	Burkina Faso, Benin, Kenya, Nigeria,	56 community members	Light shed on psychosocial challenges faced by sexual minority youth and identified both rhetoric, stereotypes, and discourse that devalue

	Rwanda, Swaziland		them and representations that counteract this symbolic violence.
Zahn R	South Africa, Namibia, Malawi, Botswana	737 MSM	A comprehensive approach with interventions at multiple levels in multiple sectors is needed to create the legal and social change necessary to address attitudes, discrimination, and violence affecting MSM.
Philip J	Trinidad and Tobago	62 HCW students	The absence of explicit negative reactions towards the homosexual HIV/AIDS patient in this study is therefore promising as it may demonstrate a tolerance of homosexuals and consequently a reduction in negative attitudes and undesirable behaviours towards homosexuals.
Cloete A	South Africa	92 MSM, 330 MSW	HIV-positive MSM reported experiencing greater social isolation and discrimination resulting from being HIV-positive, including loss of housing or employment due to their HIV status.
Padilla M	Dominican Republic	72 MSM	The participants in this study experienced significant social stigma due to their violation of norms of sexual behaviour and modes of work.

Overview of the stigma reduction interventions

Several community-level efforts have been tested and a few interventions at the organizational-level have been studied while individual-level interventions remained the most common. Interventions targeting multiple socio-ecological levels start to emerge (42).

The integrated stigma mitigation intervention

One study from Senegal evaluates the impact of the 3-tiered integrated stigma mitigation interventions (ISMIs) approach to optimizing HIV service delivery for MSM and FSW. This intervention was designed to be delivered in tiers: a) To increase participants in prevention system: a community intervention, based on peer based approach, peer-led groups sessions, that targets perceived stigma; b) to reinforce cultural and clinical competency a clinical intervention targeting enacted stigma in the health care setting; c) and a post clinical, web-based referral system intervention aiming to increase diffusion of key population-friendly services and mitigate perceived stigma (43).

The MSM-appropriate services and training program

In Kenya, the MSM-Appropriate Services and Training (MAST) consisted of eight self-administered modules delivered via computer and involved group discussions to facilitate peer support among HCPs for providing appropriate and non-judgmental HIV and STI services to MSM. After completing the training, HCPs described continued improvements in their ability to provide service in a non-stigmatizing way to MSM. In addition, four recommendations were identified: 1) expanding the reach of MSM sensitivity training across the medical education continuum; 2) establishing guidelines to manage sexually transmitted anal infections; 3) promoting legal and policy reforms to support integration of MSM-appropriate services into healthcare; and 4) including MSM information in national reporting tools for HIV services (44).

The combination HIV prevention intervention program (CHPI)

A peer-based CHPI program to target individual, social, and structural risks for HIV was developed for MSM in Malawi. It was developed to target three key levels of influence: individual, healthcare, and community. It consisted in outreach and education by peer educators based on an adapted curriculum, intensive training of HCPs and capacity building to improve the community penetration of the prevention program (45). With some limitations reported, changes in group-level sexual risk behaviors were noted, access to peer educators and engagement in CHPI provided a mechanism through which MSM were able to obtain condoms and lubricants and a number of health sector trainings have been developed to inform health care workers about health needs and HIV risks among MSM and reduce stigmatization of MSM (45).

The SPEND model

The processes of the SPEND model include Safe treatment for sexually transmissible infections (STIs) and HIV; Pharmacy sites for treatment of STIs in countries where pharmacies and drug stores are the source of medical advice and treatment; Education in sexual health issues for health professionals to reduce discrimination against MSM patients; Navigation for patients who have HIV and are rejected or discriminated against for treatment; and Discrimination reduction through educating potential leaders in tertiary education in issues of human sexuality. From a summary of empirical evidence from qualitative and quantitative studies, this model is provided as a proximal prototype to begin to conceptualize the steps that can be taken to introduce programs that begin to address provision of sexual health services to MSM in hostile climates (46).

The shikamana intervention

To design a targeted, culturally appropriate intervention to promote care engagement and antiretroviral therapy (ART) adherence for MSM in coastal Kenya, the shikamana intervention was tested from a small pilot study and the result showed its safety, feasibility, and acceptability. It combined modified Next-Step Counselling by trained providers, support from a trained peer navigator, and tailored use of SMS messaging, phone calls, and discrete pill carriers. Providers, including counsellors and clinicians, work together with peer navigators as a case management team (47).

The Ukwazana program

This is a description of the complex ways volunteer outreach workers can frame their engagement with a community-based HIV prevention program for MSM. Drawing on research conducted during one program in Cape Town called Ukwazana, it begins by exploring limitations towards MSM participation with program facilitators (namely previous feelings of mistrust and community homophobia) and strategies developed to offset these concerns. It then considers how great care must also be taken to appreciate how volunteers from marginalized groups can frame training as a key condition for participation. To understand this, it is therefore necessary for facilitators to acknowledge a number of additional concerns. These include community status, a lack of bonding social capital between volunteers and a highly developed form of critical consciousness by volunteers regarding HIV prevention possibilities. The authors therefore suggest that effort to initially engage marginalized communities must also be met with effort to understand the complex ways volunteers relate to other MSM and to each other (48).

The MSM-Appropriate services and training

This was an online education program on treatment of MSM patients, developed specifically for HCW with a clinical role, such as clinicians and nurse counsellors. It consisted of eight self-administered modules delivered via computer and involved group discussions to facilitate peer support among HCW for providing appropriate and non-judgmental HIV and STI services to MSM patients. An initial evaluation of the program was then conducted and the findings showed that at three months post-training, more HCW had acceptable levels of knowledge of MSM sexual health issues and lower levels of homophobic attitudes compared to baseline; effects were strongest among HCW with high homophobia scores at baseline. Several limitations were also mentioned (44).

Table 5. Summary of interventions studies

1st Author	Country	sample size	Main findings
Lyons CE	Senegal	NS	Need for stigma mitigation interventions, combined with enhanced linkage and retention to optimize HIV treatment.
Ross MW	Tanzania	300 MSM	The SPEND model include Safe treatment; Pharmacy sites for advice and treatment; Education to reduce discrimination against MSM; Navigation for patients who have HIV and are rejected or discriminated; and Discrimination reduction through educating potential leaders.
Van der Elst EM	Kenya	74 HCW	After completing the programme, HCWs expressed greater acknowledgement of MSM patients in their clinics, endorsed the need to treat MSM patients with high professional standards and demonstrated sophisticated awareness of the social and behavioural risks for HIV among MSM
Tucker A	South Africa	316 MSM	HIV prevention programs aimed at sexual minority groups should be mindful of potentially complex

			relationships between social stigmas such as homophobia and sexual risk-taking behaviour.
Van der Elst EM	Kenya	HCW	Four additional recommendations for improving MSM healthcare services were identified: 1) MSM sensitivity training across the medical education continuum; 2) guidelines to manage sexually transmitted anal infections; 3) promoting legal and policy reforms; and 4) including MSM information in national reporting tools for HIV services.
Wirtz AL	Malawi	8 MSM, 5 HCW	Results highlight disclosure fears among MSM and, among providers, a lack of awareness and self-efficacy to provide care in the face of limited information and political support.

3.1.2.5 Discussion

Although more research is needed, emerging evidence indicates that stigma meets all of the criteria to be considered as a fundamental barrier to prevention and treatment of HIV in the MSM population. The large volume of information reviewed and comprehensiveness of this review provided wide scope, but limited the ability to delve into specific details on particular aspects of stigma scale measurement and provider-targeted interventions. Critical challenges and gaps remain which are impeding the identification of effective stigma-reduction strategies that can be implemented on a larger scale (42). While clinical and community level interventions remained the most common, some community-level efforts have been tested in small groups and a few interventions at the organizational-level have been planned, realized and studied. HIV prevention programs aimed at sexual minority groups should be mindful of potentially complex relationships between social stigmas such as homophobia and sexual risk-taking behavior (49).

Opinions about sexuality and homosexuality comprise part of the structural factors that influence a country's response to its HIV epidemic. Based on such understanding, public messaging, communications and educational campaigns can be reshaped and targeted more effectively for the elimination of stigma and discrimination, resulting in a more effective, efficient, equitable and acceptable HIV response (37). Interventions including "safe" spaces for MSM to be educated and to obtain information in a is very crucial in societies where MSM are victims (25).

Given low levels of knowledge observed about risks associated with receptive anal intercourse, providing systematic education about the risks associated with unprotected anal intercourse represents an effective starting point (50). Supportive policy environments and prioritized HIV prevention programs for marginalized populations are vital to optimize health outcomes in key populations at high risk for HIV acquisition and transmission (51). Developing effective HIV-prevention strategies requires careful dialogue with vulnerable groups and greater flexibility for context-specific implementation rather than a one-size-fits-all conceptualization of human rights (9).

Educating the general population about the role of MSM in society and their specific health needs via the media can be a key to building mutual trust between MSM and health care providers. There still remain vital questions surrounding exactly what education needs to be provided, who is responsible or best positioned to provide such education, and how knowledge should be disseminated (32).

Arrests and convictions under laws relevant to being MSM have a strong negative association with access to HIV prevention and care services (53). In addition, lack of structural support from administrators and policy makers was seen as an impediment to improving access (54). MSM also faced economic challenges that are often seen as a consequence of their social ostracization, which resulted in limited social support, an interrupted education, and reduced earning power (48,55).

A further reflection needs to be done on the weakness between homosexuality and the attention given by healthcare professional and healthcare students. The MSM population experience difficulties engaging in care and disclose their behaviours and adhere due to the embarrassing situations when expressing their homosexuality/bisexuality, due to the homophobia present in professionals. Important revisions of curricula to introduce this topic in health sciences undergraduate's curricula; conducting training with already working professionals; monitoring the capacity-building interventions are needed. Although they were some limitations, data reinforce the need for stigma mitigation interventions to be combined with enhanced linkage and retention to HIV care and treatment to optimize HIV outcomes among MSM.

Stigma measurement tools continue to be an important issue. The lack of standardized measurement tools for stigma and discrimination greatly limits our way to design and judge which strategies work the best for addressing the various stigma domains or targeting different socio-ecological levels. The development of validated measures assessing each domain of the stigmatization process must be a priority in order to shift with programmatic efforts and/or structural interventions (42). However, this review found a few validated scales created for measuring MSM-associated stigma and some others adapted for the studies but not validated. The availability of tested stigma-reduction tools and approaches need to be improved. What is also needed is the political will and resources to support and scale up stigma reduction activities throughout health care settings.

Important limitations of this analysis need to be highlighted. The life sciences and biomedical literature were reviewed but other relevant sources, particularly relating to socio-anthropological, policy, and legal analyses, may not have been captured. Studies from Africa and The Caribbean only were reviewed in order to find a description and interventions that came from regions with similar cultural and ethnic background. Studies from PubMed only were reviewed and quality was not assessed. Further systematic review on interventions specifically is needed in order to compare and evaluate them so more lessons can be learned.

Conclusion

Our hope is that within the next years, more interventions will be developed, tested and implemented and countries will be collecting programmatic data demonstrating the impact of stigma and discrimination reduction on HIV prevention and care outcomes in MSM population. Considering the negative impact of stigma on individual health and health systems results, it is an evidence that health care stakeholders cannot afford inaction any longer. Furthermore, messages for key populations should be complemented by producing messages for the wider "general" population as part of a comprehensive HIV response to reduce stigma and discrimination.

3.1.2.6 References

1.   Beck, E. J. *et al.* Attitudes towards homosexuals in seven Caribbean countries: implications for an effective HIV response. *AIDS Care* **29,** 1557–1566 (2017).

2.   Lebouché, B. & Levy, J. J. Nouveaux traitements et indétectabilité du VIH. Un risque dans la relation médecin-patient ? *Médecine et Maladies Infectieuses* **39,** (2009).

3.   Unaids   Factsheet.   Available   at: http://www.unaids.org/sites/default/files/media_asset/UNAIDS_FactSheet_en.pdf. (Accessed: 13th March 2021)

4.   Mahajan, A. P. *et al.* Stigma in the HIV/AIDS epidemic: a review of the literature and recommendations for the way forward. *AIDS* **22,** (2008).

5.   Smit, P. J. *et al.* HIV-related stigma within communities of gay men: a literature review. *AIDS Care* **24,** 405–412 (2011).

6.   Amirkhanian, Y. A. Social Networks, Sexual Networks and HIV Risk in Men Who Have Sex with Men. *Current HIV/AIDS Reports* **11,** 81–92 (2014).

7.   Cáceres, C. F. HIV among gay and other men who have sex with men in Latin America and the Caribbean: a hidden epidemic?*. *AIDS* **16,** (2002).

8.   Papworth, E. *et al.* Epidemiology of HIV among female sex workers, their clients, men who have sex with men and people who inject drugs in West and Central Africa. *Journal of the International AIDS Society* **16,** 18751 (2013).

9.   Muzyamba, C., Broaddus, E. & Campbell, C. "You cannot eat rights": a qualitative study of views by Zambian HIV-vulnerable women, youth and MSM on human rights as public health tools. *BMC International Health and Human Rights* **15,** (2015).

10.   Cloete, A., Simbayi, L. C., Kalichman, S. C., Strebel, A. & Henda, N. Stigma and discrimination experiences of HIV-positive men who have sex with men in Cape Town, South Africa. *AIDS Care* **20,** 1105–1110 (2008).

11.   Fay, H. *et al.* Stigma, Health Care Access, and HIV Knowledge Among Men Who Have Sex With Men in Malawi, Namibia, and Botswana. *AIDS and Behavior* **15,** 1088–1097 (2010).

12.   Baral, S., Sifakis, F., Cleghorn, F. & Beyrer, C. Elevated Risk for HIV Infection among Men Who Have Sex with Men in Low- and Middle-Income Countries 2000–2006: A Systematic Review. *PLoS Medicine* **4,** (2007).

13.   Polsky, H. W. Book Review: Stigma: Notes on the Management of Spoiled Identity. *Social Casework* **45,** 357–358 (1964).

14.   Hightow-Weidman, L. *et al.* Exploring the HIV continuum of care among young black MSM. *PLOS ONE* **12,** (2017).

15.   MacLean, R. Resources to address stigma related to sexuality, substance use and sexually transmitted and blood-borne infections. *Canada Communicable Disease Report* **44,** 62–67 (2018).

16.   Baxter, C. The Dilemma of Difference: A Multidisciplinary View of Stigma. *Disability, Handicap & Society* **2,** 298–300 (1987).

17.   Link, B. G. & Phelan, J. C. Conceptualizing Stigma. *Annual Review of Sociology* **27,** 363–385 (2001).

18.   Weiss, M. G., Ramakrishna, J. & Somma, D. Health-related stigma: Rethinking concepts and interventions 1. *Psychology, Health & Medicine* **11,** 277–287 (2006).

19.   Goffman, E. & Kihm, A. *Stigmate: les usages sociaux des handicaps*. (Les Éditions de minuit, 2015).

20.   Fitzgerald-Husek, A. *et al.* Measuring stigma affecting sex workers (SW) and men who have sex with men (MSM): A systematic review. *PLOS ONE* **12,** (2017).

21.   2016 United Nations Political Declaration on Ending AIDS sets world on the Fast-Track to end the epidemic by 2030. *UNAIDS Viet Nam 2016 United Nations Political Declaration on Ending AIDS sets world on the FastTrack to end the epidemic by 2030 Comments* Available at: https://unaids.org.vn/2016-united-nations-political-declaration-ending-aids-sets-world-fast-track-end-epidemic-2030/. (Accessed: 13th March 2021)

22.   Winskell, K. & Sabben, G. Sexual stigma and symbolic violence experienced, enacted, and counteracted in young Africans' writing about same-sex attraction. *Social Science & Medicine* **161,** 143–150 (2016).

23.   Larsson, M., Mohamed Shio, J., Ross, M. W. & Agardh, A. Acting within an increasingly confined space: A qualitative study of sexual behaviours and healthcare needs among men who have sex with men in a provincial Tanzanian city. *PLOS ONE* **12,** (2017).

24.   Logie, C. H. *et al.* Social–ecological factors associated with HIV infection among men who have sex with men in Jamaica. *International Journal of STD & AIDS* **29,** 80–88 (2017).

25.   Sithole, B. HIV prevention needs for men who have sex with men in Swaziland. *African Journal of AIDS Research* **16,**315–320 (2017).

26.   Ruiseñor-Escudero, H. *et al.* Using a social ecological framework to characterize the correlates of HIV among men who have sex with men in Lomé, Togo. *AIDS Care* **29,** 1169–1177 (2017).

27.   Brown, C. A. *et al.* Characterizing the Individual, Social, and Structural Determinants of Condom Use Among Men Who Have Sex with Men in Swaziland. *AIDS Research and Human Retroviruses* **32,** 539–546 (2016).

28.   Padilla, M. *et al.* Stigma, social inequality, and HIV risk disclosure among Dominican male sex workers. *Social Science & Medicine* **67,** 380–388 (2008).

29.   Poteat, T. *et al.* HIV prevalence and behavioral and psychosocial factors among transgender women and cisgender men who have sex with men in 8 African countries: A cross-sectional analysis. *PLOS Medicine* **14,** (2017).

30.   Taegtmeyer, M. *et al.* Challenges in Providing Counselling to MSM in Highly Stigmatized Contexts: Results of a Qualitative Study from Kenya. *PLoS ONE* **8,** (2013).

31.   van Rooyen, H. *et al.* What are the constraints and opportunities for HIVST scale-up in Africa? Evidence from Kenya, Malawi and South Africa. *Journal of the International AIDS Society* **18,** 19445 (2015).

32.   Kushwaha, S. *et al.* "But the moment they find out that you are MSM…": a qualitative investigation of HIV prevention experiences among men who have sex with men (MSM) in Ghana's health care system. *BMC Public Health* **17,**(2017).

33.   Logie, C. H. *et al.* Social–ecological factors associated with HIV infection among men who have sex with men in Jamaica. *International Journal of STD & AIDS* **29,** 80–88 (2017).

34.   Shangani, S. *et al.* Factors associated with HIV testing among men who have sex with men in Western Kenya: a cross-sectional study. *International Journal of STD & AIDS* **28,** 179–187 (2016).

35.   Wanyenze, R. K. *et al.* "If You Tell People That You Had Sex with a Fellow Man, It Is Hard to Be Helped and Treated": Barriers and Opportunities for Increasing Access to HIV Services among Men Who Have Sex with Men in Uganda. *PLOS ONE* **11,** (2016).

36.   Micheni, M. *et al.* Health Provider Views on Improving Antiretroviral Therapy Adherence Among Men Who Have Sex with Men in Coastal Kenya. *AIDS Patient Care and STDs* **31,** 113–121 (2017).

37.   Beck, E. J. *et al.* Attitudes towards homosexuals in seven Caribbean countries: implications for an effective HIV response. *AIDS Care* **29,** 1557–1566 (2017).

38.   Schwartz, S. R. *et al.* The immediate effect of the Same-Sex Marriage Prohibition Act on stigma, discrimination, and engagement on HIV prevention and treatment services in men who have sex with men in Nigeria: analysis of prospective data from the TRUST cohort. *The Lancet HIV* **2,** (2015).

39.   Scheibe, A. *et al.* Finding solid ground: law enforcement, key populations and their health and rights in South Africa. *Journal of the International AIDS Society* **19,** 20872 (2016).

40.   Duvall, S. *et al.* Assessment of Policy and Access to HIV Prevention, Care, and Treatment Services for Men Who Have Sex With Men and for Sex Workers in Burkina Faso and Togo. *JAIDS Journal of Acquired Immune Deficiency Syndromes* **68,** (2015).

41.   Andrinopoulos, K., Figueroa, J. P., Kerrigan, D. & Ellen, J. M. Homophobia, stigma and HIV in Jamaican prisons. *Culture, Health & Sexuality* **13,** 187–200 (2011).

42.   Stangl, A. L., Lloyd, J. K., Brady, L. M., Holland, C. E. & Baral, S. A systematic review of interventions to reduce HIV-related stigma and discrimination from 2002 to 2013: how far have we come? *Journal of the International AIDS Society* **16,** 18734 (2013).

43.   Lyons, C. E. *et al.* Potential Impact of Integrated Stigma Mitigation Interventions in Improving HIV/AIDS Service Delivery and Uptake for Key Populations in Senegal. *JAIDS Journal of Acquired Immune Deficiency Syndromes* **74,**(2017).

44.   van der Elst, E. M. *et al.* The green shoots of a novel training programme: progress and identified key actions to providing services to MSM at Kenyan health facilities. *Journal of the International AIDS Society* **18,** 20226 (2015).

45.   Wirtz, A. L. *et al.* Feasibility of a Combination HIV Prevention Program for Men Who Have Sex With Men in Blantyre, Malawi. *JAIDS Journal of Acquired Immune Deficiency Syndromes* **70,** 155–162 (2015).

46.   Ross, M. W. *et al.* Health care in a homophobic climate: the SPEND model for providing sexual health services to men who have sex with men where their health and human rights are compromised. *Global Health Action* **8,** 26096 (2015).

47.   Graham, S. M. *et al.* Development and pilot testing of an intervention to promote care engagement and adherence among HIV-positive Kenyan MSM. *AIDS* **29,** (2015).

48.   Tucker, A., de Swardt, G., Struthers, H. & McIntyre, J. Understanding the Needs of Township Men Who have Sex with Men (MSM) Health Outreach Workers: Exploring the Interplay Between Volunteer Training, Social Capital and Critical Consciousness. *AIDS and Behavior* **17,** 33–42 (2012).

49.   Tucker, A. *et al.* Homophobic stigma, depression, self-efficacy and unprotected anal intercourse for peri-urban township men who have sex with men in Cape Town, South Africa: a cross-sectional association model. *AIDS Care* **26,** 882–889 (2013).

50.   Mason, K. *et al.* A Cross-Sectional Analysis of Population Demographics, HIV Knowledge and Risk Behaviors, and Prevalence and Associations of HIV Among Men Who Have Sex with Men in the Gambia. *AIDS Research and Human Retroviruses* **29,** 1547–1552 (2013).

51.   Zahn, R. *et al.* Human Rights Violations among Men Who Have Sex with Men in Southern Africa: Comparisons between Legal Contexts. *PLOS ONE* **11,** (2016).

52.   Muzyamba, C., Broaddus, E. & Campbell, C. "You cannot eat rights": a qualitative study of views by Zambian HIV-vulnerable women, youth and MSM on human rights as public health tools. *BMC International Health and Human Rights* **15,** (2015).

53.   Santos, G.-M., Makofane, K., Arreola, S., Do, T. & Ayala, G. Reductions in access to HIV prevention and care services are associated with arrest and convictions in a global survey of men who have sex with men. *Sexually Transmitted Infections* **93,** 62–64 (2016).

54.   Kennedy, C. E. *et al.* "They are human beings, they are Swazi": intersecting stigmas and the positive health, dignity and prevention needs of HIV-positive men who have sex with men in Swaziland. *Journal of the International AIDS Society* **16,** 18749 (2013).

55.   Risher, K. *et al.* Sexual stigma and discrimination as barriers to seeking appropriate healthcare among men who have sex with men in Swaziland. *Journal of the International AIDS Society* **16,** 18715 (2013).

Presentation of the study 3:

As the two previous studies explored the role of stigma on the steps of the continuum from identification to undetectable viral load. The second one showed the importance of the continuum both as an individual-level tool to assess care outcomes, as well as a population-level framework to analyze the proportion of MSM who are engaged in each successive step. It highlighted the way this tool helps policymakers and service providers to better pinpoint where gaps might exist and develop strategies to better support MSM to achieve the treatment goal of viral suppression.

An overwhelming body of clinical evidence has firmly established the HIV Undetectable=Untransmissible, or U=U meaning that MSM who achieve and maintain an undetectable viral load cannot sexually transmit the virus to others. U=U represents the ultimate goal of the Continuum. To achieve this goal, all stakeholders, including care givers, must work towards the full implementation of the strategies. Attitudes of care givers towards MSM play a significant role on retention in care and medical outcomes. As MSM are, sometimes, subject to layers of bias, their perception of prejudice or negative attitude is associated with lower healthcare quality, reduced enrolment, treatment adherence and poor medical outcomes, impeding the U=U. The next study assessed the attitudes that medical students harbour toward MSM infected with HIV to better understand the extent to which stigma and other factors may impair actual and future healthcare delivery to MSM patients and to explore suggestions of opportunities for making such services more welcoming and socially accountable regarding the Haitian context.

Study 3

Title: Attitudes of medical students towards men who have sex with men living with HIV: implications for social accountability

Running Head: Attitudes of medical students towards MSM

Willy Dunbar, MD[1, 2, 3 §], Marie Colette Alcide Jean-Pierre, MD[3, 4], Christian Raccurt, MD[3], Jean William Pape, MD[2], Yves Coppieters, PhD[1]

1 Health Systems and Policies - International Health, School of Public Health, Université libre de Bruxelles (ULB), Brussels, Belgium
2 Haitian Study Group for Kaposi's Sarcoma and Opportunistic Infections (GHESKIO), Port-au-Prince, Haiti
3 Faculty of Health Sciences, Quisqueya University, Port-au-Prince, Haiti
4 Infectious Diseases Department, Saint-Camille Hospital, Port-au-Prince, Haiti

[§] Corresponding author: Willy Dunbar

Citation:
Dunbar W, Alcide C, Raccurt C, Pape JW, Coppieters Y. Attitudes of medical students towards men who have sex with men living with HIV: implications for social accountability. Int J Med Educ. 2020 Oct 23;11:233-239. doi: 10.5116/ijme.5f87.39c2. PMID: 33099520; PMCID: PMC7882130.

International Journal of Medical Education. 2020;11:233-239
ISSN: 2042-6372
DOI: 10.5116/ijme.5f87.39c2

Attitudes of medical students towards men who have sex with men living with HIV: implications for social accountability

Willy Dunbar[1], Marie Colette Alcide Jean-Pierre[2], Christian Raccurt[2], Jean William Pape[3], Yves Coppieters[1]

[1]Health Systems and Policies, International Health, School of Public Health, Université libre de Bruxelles (ULB), Brussels, Belgium
[2]Faculty of Health Sciences, Quisqueya University, Port-au-Prince, Haiti
[3]Haitian Study Group for Kaposi's Sarcoma and Opportunistic Infections (GHESKIO), Port-au-Prince, Haiti

Correspondence: Willy Dunbar, École de Santé Publique, Campus Erasme - Bâtiment A, Route de Lennik 808 - CP591, Bruxelles, 1070, Belgium. Email: wdunbar@ulb.ac.be

Accepted: October 14, 2020

receive equitable care, the moral responsibility of healthcare professionals, their perception of health disparities and the HIV global risk reduction. Participants pointed out that the medical education curriculum did not consider sexual health and specificities of sexual minorities and suggested a more inclusive and socially accountable training based on equity and quality.

Conclusions: The students expressed favourable attitudes regarding health services to Men who have Sex with Men even though some layered stigmatizing attitudes emerged through the discussions. They all lacked skills on how to handle health specificities of sexual minorities. These findings recommend a revision of the medical education curriculum in regard to social accountability principles.

Keywords: Haiti, HIV, men who have sex with men, medical student, social accountability

Introduction

Advances in scientific understanding of HIV prevention and treatment by the global health community, government and civil society organizations have made it possible to control the epidemic.[1] To achieve the goal of ending HIV by 2030, targets have been set by the United Nations for HIV diagnosis and care continuum. The 95-95-95 goals aim for 95% of individuals infected with HIV to be aware of their status, 95% of those diagnosed to initiate antiretroviral (ARV) treatment, and 95% of those on ARVs to have undetectable viral loads.[2] While this goal has been set, in 2018, key populations (KP) and their sexual partners accounted for 54% of new HIV infections globally, and among the KP, Men who have Sex with Men (MSM) accounted for 17%.[3] In Haiti, a country of the Caribbean, which is the most affected region after Africa, prevention and treatment strategies implemented in collaboration with international organizations and donors have contributed to reducing the national HIV prevalence from 6.2% in 1993 to 2% in 2018. However, according to a survey conducted and published by the United Nations, the HIV prevalence among MSM was 18.2% in 2017, making them the most underserved population in terms of HIV prevention and care.[4-6]

233

In order to fulfil the targets to properly include and retain MSM in the continuum of care, attitudes of caregivers play a critical role. As MSM are at an increased risk for HIV and continue to bear a disproportional burden of the infection, many barriers prevent or limit their access to proper care.[7] Among the barriers to accessing healthcare, stigma, discrimination and confidentiality remain major concerns.[8] Indeed, despite many efforts that are being made to improve the management of HIV, stigma remains a challenging issue.[9] Therefore, as the response to the epidemic continues to grow, stigma continues to hamper the healthcare services, and people living with HIV (PLHIV) are often perceived as having socially despised behaviours.[10-12]

Previous studies conducted in several settings have reported suboptimal uptake of services among MSM; these findings have been attributed to a lack of trust and non-responsiveness to the health needs of MSM on the part of the providers.[8,13] HIV sometimes evoke irrational emotions and fears, and the degree of bias perceived by patients in healthcare settings depends on the provider's knowledge about HIV, experience working with PLHIV and HIV-related fears.[14,15] Medical students represent the next generation of clinicians responsible for HIV care efforts, and they often reflect attitudes held in their society and community of practice.[16] Studies assessing attitudes of medical students towards MSM have also shown expression of discomfort with the behaviour of gay men and the prevalence of reluctance to provide proper medical care.[17,18] As MSM are subjected to layers of bias, their perception of negative attitudes is associated with reduced enrolment, reduced treatment adherence and poor medical outcomes.[19,20] In this regard, medical education and services should be directed towards eliminating the concerns and health priorities of the society and take into account the complexity and changing expectations of health systems, hence the implications of the social accountability concept advocating for equity, quality, relevance and effectiveness.[21] Thus, socially accountable training to understand the needs and willingness of providing care for those at highest risk is critical to ensuring that efforts at HIV detection, linkage to HIV care and retention are successful.

The extents to which MSM are stigmatized by health care providers and the attitudes of medical students towards MSM have been investigated in several contexts, yet to the best of our knowledge, no studies have focused on those issues in Haiti.[18,22,23] The aims of this study were firstly, to assess the attitudes that medical students harbour towards MSM and better understand the extent to which stigma and other factors may impair actual and future healthcare, and secondly, to explore suggestions of opportunities for making such services socially accountable. We chose to focus on MSM because the social climate of stigma, fear of discrimination and lack of knowledge among health care providers are part of the reasons why this group is the most

marginalized and still left behind by the health systems, putting them at increased risk of HIV.[24]

Methods

Study design

We utilized a qualitative study design by using a grounded theory approach regarding the context of Haiti.[25] We sought to assess the attitude of medical students towards MSM living with HIV based on an inductive approach, which provided the framework for data analysis.[26,27]

Study setting

Quisqueya University School of Health Sciences is a medical school located in Port-au-Prince, the capital city of Haiti. As the largest private university, the school of Health Sciences comprises 800 students originating from all administrative departments of the country. The six-year medical programme is divided into two-year basic sciences and four-year clinical sciences in partnership with associated academic hospitals located not only in the capital city but also in several rural and urban regions of the country ensuring practice through various cultures and contexts. The programme also entails clinical placements in infectious diseases and HIV settings where students work under the supervision of clinical tutors. As part of the social accountability reform process for accreditation renewal, efforts are being made to have a substantial basic science, clinical, and epidemiological community-oriented research activity within the university and associated academic hospitals.

Participants and data collection

We used purposive sampling to select the research participants, which comprised 11 males and 11 females. Ages of the participants vary from 23 to 26 years; 20 of them identified themselves as Christians (Catholic and Protestants), and two did not mention their religion. The participants were in their final step of the clinical sciences programme and already spent three years in clinical placement at the associated academic hospitals. Among them, 17 indicated that they have already provided care for MSM during their clerkships in HIV facilities. For those who indicated that they had never served any MSM and therefore did not have any experience to share, we asked them to imagine what would happen if they were to take care of MSM. Eligibility was met if they were registered in the final year and had clinical training and practice in providing care to PLHIV. In order to ensure maximum variation, we managed to elicit views from diverse categories of students with different ages, sex, city of origin and religious beliefs.

The interview guide was made in accordance with the study objectives. The questions were open-ended, with probes used to explore points raised by interviewees or for clarification where more information was required. Data was collected through in-depth interviews from the 22 participants selected. We explored their personal views on PLHIV in general, their attitudes regarding MSM living with HIV, their willingness to provide care for them, their experiences with MSM in the clinical settings, and suggestions towards provision of sexual healthcare targeting and appropriate for MSM. The interview guide was available depending on the language preference of the interviewee (French or Haitian Creole). All participants preferred to be interviewed in Haitian Creole, but some responses were also provided in French; interviews lasted between 35 to 55 minutes. We allowed enough time with participants to ensure that adequate data were collected during the interview and continued the process until we reached saturation. Participants were free to ask questions on issues they felt were not clear to them. Permission was obtained to audio record the interviews. The interviewer was ready to take notes where an audio recording would have been declined. Ethical approval for the study was obtained from the Haitian Group for the Study of Kaposi's Sarcoma and Opportunistic Infections' human right committee and the Cornell University Weil Medical College's Research Ethics Board. Prior to interviewing, the study purpose and expectations of involvement were explained in Haitian Creole to the participants. We obtained oral and written informed consent from all participants. Data were stored in a secure place, and the anonymity was maintained through de-identification.

Data analysis

Recorded interviews were transcribed verbatim. We reviewed the transcribed data to ensure understanding and then compared these transcripts with the original audio recordings for accuracy. The primary author read and reviewed the transcripts multiple times and selected one transcript for the initial open coding. To validate the coding process, a clean copy of the same transcript was de-identified and given to another experienced qualitative researcher to conduct a separate independent open coding which was later verified by co-authors. The primary author assessed both coding outputs and came up with one generic coding frame for indexing the rest of the codes. Relationships and comparisons between themes were generated from the coding frame in an iterative process. This ensured that attention was given for consistent patterns within the data focusing on similarities and differences on responses given by participants to aid analysis and interpretation. Our approach to data analysis was based on the thematic analysis in line with the study aim.

Four techniques were used to support the trustworthiness of the work: credibility, dependability, conformability and transferability.[28,29] Prior to data collection and in order to understand the contextual factors relating to the HIV care continuum for MSM, three meetings and two participant observation sessions were held with MSM patients, HIV caregivers and medical students at two HIV-associated academic centres and at the main campus of the Université Quisqueya. Credibility was established by selecting in-depth interview method for the data collection and by the researcher who conducted the interviews being familiar with the context. Dependability was established by describing the data analysis in detail and providing direct citations to reveal the basis from which the analysis was conducted. The citations used in this article were translated from Haitian Creole into English with the help of a translator, to maintain accuracy and context as much as possible. The conformability and consistency of the analysis were established by holding meetings for the authors to discuss preliminary findings, emerging codes and themes until a consensus was reached. To enhance the transferability of the findings, a description of the context, selection and demographics of participants, data collection and process of analysis is provided to enable the reader determine whether the results of this study are transferable to another context.

Results

The study findings have been grouped by themes. Thus, we present the themes and supporting quotations to illustrate the main findings.

Willingness to provide care to MSM infected with HIV All students indicated that they were or would be comfortable serving MSM, although a few of them expressed some level of discomfort. They expressed their willingness to provide MSM with comprehensive HIV care. Their expressions were based on the right for MSM to receive care, the moral responsibility of healthcare professionals and the perceived health disparities regarding MSM in the population.

Right to receive comprehensive care

The participants of the study stated that every human being has the right to receive adequate healthcare services regardless of their sexual practices and sexual orientation. They expressed their readiness to address MSM's medical issues unreservedly.

> *"...MSMs are human beings so they deserve and have the right to good treatment...we are the future of the health society in this country and we need to be ready to consider everyone as equal..."* [Student 3, male, 23 years old]

Moral responsibility

Participants indicated that in their capacity as students soon-to-be graduated, taking care of MSM is a moral duty in regard to the Hippocratic Oath.

> *"... We will have Hippocrates' oath and diploma ceremony so we'll have to respect our promise..."* [Student 9, female, 23 years old]

Thus, they expressed their compliance to provide MSM with services in much the same way as they would for other patients and maintain the expected level of confidentiality.

> *"I don't think we have the choice; I choose to study medicine so I can take care of sick people... straight or gay, they need us...we are here to listen and to understand them..."* [Student 16, male, 23 years old]

Perception of health disparities

Stigma from healthcare professionals was identified by the participants as a reason why MSM may be reluctant to take up healthcare services. Participants agreed that this is one of the reasons why they have a responsibility to provide care without discrimination.

> "...We cannot let them apart because they are already neglected by some doctors and nurses... I saw a nurse talking really bad to a boy because he was acting and talking like a girl..." [Student 13, female, 24 years old]

HIV risk reduction

Some participants expressed their concerns about the high risk of HIV infection among MSM, who are perceived as a bridge through which HIV is spread to the general population. Thus, they expressed their willingness to take care of them in order to reduce this risk.

> "...gay men have greater risk to get HIV and they have sex with girls too; that's like a [cycle]. If we let them out, the epidemic will become very important again..." [Student 16, male, 23 years old]

Layered stigma and lack of specific skills to provide MSM with comprehensive HIV care

Evidence from studies suggests that MSM-related training reduces homophobic sentiments from health care providers.[30] We asked the participants if their training has provided them with sexual health knowledge to address MSM specificities.

Patient-provider misunderstanding

The findings revealed that medical education curriculum does not consider MSM specificities. Students explicitly expressed their limitations in relation to health of sexual minorities. Some of them explained that their professors and clinical instructors do not address MSM particularities and went further by explaining some stigmatizing attitudes they had noted from them.

> "... I don't think we learn much because some professors laugh when we bring discussions about gay. They don't like talking about them; it's a sensitive topic..." [Student 8, male, 24 years old]

Although they all agreed that taking care of MSM is an obligation, some male participants expressed some level of discomfort.

> "...I don't mind take care of them but they have to respect me. Gay people are too open. In the hospital they called me...told stories and touching me...I can't have contact with them..." [Student 10, male, 24 years old]

They affirmed that MSM could try to harass them during medical examination. Moreover, some students think that taking care of not only MSM but also any PLHIV require specific protection equipment like gloves and masks. These sentiments suggest a lack of medical and communication skills in HIV and sexual health.

> "I called a nurse to assist me... so he doesn't touch me...sincerely I was afraid staying alone with him in the examination room...sometimes they are violent..." [Student 2, female, 24 years old]

Layered stigma about homosexuality

Some students expressed a level of discomfort when it comes to holding discussions with MSM about sexual relationships.

> "I would feel uncomfortable asking questions about their private life. I don't need to know their private life, it's disgusting. This is why they are sick..." [Student 14, male, 26 years old]

When we probed further about the feeling of discomfort, some of them expressed their disagreement of same-sex relationship and their disposition to try to convince MSM to leave such practice.

> "...This is a sin. God doesn't like that, so as a doctor I can try to convince them to leave such life..." [Student 10, male, 24 years old]

These findings suggest the need to continue questioning their ability to properly address sexual health issues and confirm the need for medical curriculum to address MSM-sensitive topics.

Implications for social accountability

Social accountability in health stems from a social contract which outlines the roles of training institutions in regard to the societies within which they are located and from where they draw their resources.[31] A socially accountable physician is one who has a deep and profound understanding of his or her community responsibilities, having been trained in the community with a view towards population health and eliminating health inequities in partnership with community members.[32]

In regard to this principle, we wanted to explore what the students would suggest to address the gap related to MSM-specific sexual health in their medical education. They expressed key ideas on how to make it more inclusive and socially accountable through the following two areas:

Inclusive medical education

Some students indicated the need for MSM-related issues and specificities in their curriculum.

> "I think a training in MSM-related care will help us understand them better" [Student 18, female, 24 years old]

They suggested classes on physical and psychological needs of sexual minorities.

> *"…We see them everywhere but we don't even know how to properly communicate on issues that may affect their health…"* [Student 16, male, 23 years old]

Non-judgmental and caring attitudes of professors

One of the solutions that the students pointed out is a change in attitude of their professors who sometimes mock MSM during classes and clinical training even if they don't agree. They went further and called for a need to train their professors.

> *"…I think our professors don't give us a chance to learn about sexual minorities' health because they don't know much about them either. If they can participate in conferences about gay men, they would probably be more tolerant in their words and attitudes during classes…"* [Student 8, male, 24 years old]

Understanding patients' needs with respect to their identity and preserving the human dignity of individuals with their multiple social identities are essential, and these findings reinforce the concept. Implications for social accountability in regards to specific health needs of MSM in Haiti stems particularly from two values: equity—which requires student learners to engage with minority groups, and quality—which promotes multi-professional and policy partners in teamwork to address major social determinants of health.[33]

What then do these findings imply for medical education in Haiti? It can enable a reflection process for medical education policymakers and healthcare professionals to analyze medical curricula, legislation and public health policies more critically while considering contextual factors which can perpetuate the cycle of social disparities. It can also help to better understand and address the social health inequalities in regard to social determinants of health. Concretely, applying the social accountability values through interventions will give visibility to stigmatized and marginalized populations such as MSM and improve the competencies of healthcare professionals to adapt their practices to the complexity of population needs and health system stakes.[34,35]

Discussion

Our study revealed three main findings: a) participants expressed their willingness to provide MSM with comprehensive healthcare; b) medical education curriculum does not consider MSM-specific sexual health and emerging layered stigma attitudes while providing comprehensive services through a discussion about same-sex relationship; and c) suggestions of a more inclusive medical education and non-judgmental, caring attitudes of professors and clinical instructors.

In this study, the majority of students were in support of adequate healthcare delivery to MSM infected with HIV. They stated that MSM has health needs like other patients and deserve access to appropriate healthcare. They reflected on their professional responsibility by referring to the Hippocratic Oath to highlight their willingness. Our findings are in line with another study conducted in Malawi, showing that medical students expressed their entire willingness to provide MSM with appropriate healthcare.[36] However, in contrast, negative attitudes towards MSM were found to be high in Malaysia and Russia.[17] Access to healthcare in some countries where MSM are not protected by law is still challenging. However, it has been proved that negative attitudes of health care providers have shifted due to the implementation of educational interventions; one of the recommendations made by the participants.[37]

Another reason for their reflection was to reduce health inequity and global HIV risk. This finding refers to the recommendations by the World Health Organization for MSM.38 Stigma is indeed perceived and experienced in healthcare settings, and anxiety about HIV status, its social consequences and confidentiality concerns are major deterrents to accessing HIV care and exacerbate health inequity among MSM. A study from Ghana supports the contribution of tailored interventions to reduce health inequity.[39] Moreover, another study from the United States demonstrated that scaling up a group of interventions targeting both health care providers and MSM like sensitization sessions and peer support are important.[40]

While students feel the obligation to provide care to MSM like any other patient, some of them would not be comfortable. Homophobia represents a major barrier to accessing HIV services among MSM.[12] They also have limited access to specialized programmes, even in comparison with people who inject drugs and sex workers.[41] While considering the fact that MSM may opt not to reveal their sexual orientation to health care providers due to these attitudes, more studies are needed to understand all forms of homophobia in clinical settings. Moreover, programmes focused on clinical interventions need to also consider human right issues.

The students clearly indicated that they did not have the requisite skills necessary to handle MSM health specificities; most of them felt that they not only needed to be clinically trained, effective communication training sessions required to be delivered to their professors. Several previous studies have documented that a lack of specific skills can affect continuum of care for MSM.[36,37,40] In contrast, other studies showed that health care providers trained in MSM specificity provide better holistic care while considering the social aspects of their lives.[30] It follows that training of health care providers will lead to skill improvement for quality of healthcare; however, efforts to shift attitudes have to consider the cultural components of the society.

By mentioning the negative attitudes of their professors, some students pointed out their role in shaping the actual and future model of care in Haitian society. In 1990, a study from the United States found that medical school professors can be a source of negativity regarding HIV positive and marginalized groups.[42] In fact, the senior doctors define and portray attitudes during the learning process, which will probably stay with future healthcare professionals throughout their career. However, participatory training methods and interventions tested by other studies showed valuable tools for changing attitudes and decreasing biases.[30]

Although the issues that MSM face are documented, gaps remain in the medical curriculum. Some countries have started incorporating MSM health in their medical curriculum, while Haiti has limited engagement with the topic. Medical students need didactic sessions to be incorporated into the curriculum so that their knowledge of how social determinants impact the health of MSM can be addressed alongside interventions and research efforts on increasing comfort and mitigating stigma.[31,33,43]

Evidence of the link between health training institutions and communities has been around for a long time; however, it is only in recent decades that social accountability of health education has become more formalized.[31] The "social contract" defines the duties of the training institutions with regard to all aspects of the societies in which they are established and where they draw their resources.[32,33] Thus, solutions and strategies that gradually stimulate the adaptation of health professions to the realities of every community, including MSM, are necessary to strengthen professional ethics for the respect of rights, duties and freedom without stigma.

This is a qualitative study that explored attitudes of medical students towards MSM living with HIV, an area clearly lacking in research. The results represent the views of a single medical student population in Haiti to a single stigmatized group; this may limit the generalisability of the study findings. However, we tried to improve external validity by selecting participants from different backgrounds and culture. Our study did not evaluate a respondent's level of practice during medical education to determine whether attitudes changed with an increased amount of experience. However, the description of acceptability to provide HIV-related health services among students as elicited in this study could be valid in another setting with similar context. Despite these limitations, participants came from different backgrounds in terms of religion and city of origin; they also practice in the same academic hospitals with students from other medical schools and share same professors and clinical instructors. By documenting the attitudes, our study provides critical insight into the extent to which stigma towards MSM living with HIV is endorsed—not only by the students but also by the professors—and highlights the need for stigma mitigation interventions.

Conclusions

This qualitative study explored the attitudes of medical students towards MSM living with HIV in Haiti. The study showed that medical students were willing to provide MSM-focused HIV care services. They recognized the right for MSM to have equal access to services as other patients and proposed intervention strategies to address MSM-specific gaps in their medical education. However, future researches are required to capture more views, experiences and propositions from not only medical students but experienced healthcare givers in order to propose socially accountable interventions targeting revision of curriculum and more equitable HIV care for MSM in Haïti. The shift from evidence to action requires synergy in the socio-centric evolution of health to enhance relevance, quality, efficiency and equity of the social accountability of medical education, as stigmatized populations and sexual minorities can no longer be kept unchecked in the era of 'Leave no one behind' for a world free of HIV.

Authors' contributions

WD, CA, CR, JWP and YC conceived the original research idea and led the design of the study. WD, CA and YC developed the protocol and the topic guide. WD, CA and YC conducted the analysis. WD and CA developed the first draft of the article. All authors oversaw the development of the article and contributed to the revisions. All authors reviewed and approved the final draft.

Acknowledgements

We thank the Université Quisqueya's administration and the Dean's office for their support and assistance and all the students for their willingness to participate in the study.

Conflicts of Interest

The authors declare that they have no conflicts of interest.

References

1. Jin H, Earnshaw V, Wickersham J, Kamarulzaman A, Desai M, John J, et al. An assessment of healthcare students' attitudes toward patients with or at high risk for HIV: implications for education and cultural competency. AIDS Care. 2014;26(10):1223-1228.

2. Zuniga J. UNAIDS 90-90-90—Opportunity in every difficulty. J Int Assoc Provid AIDS Care. 2018;17:1-2.

3. United Nations. A United Nations update on the global AIDS epidemic. Population and Development Review. 2018;44(1):189-191.

4. Rouzier V, Farmer P, Pape J, Jerome J, Van Onacker J, Morose W, et al. Factors impacting the provision of antiretroviral therapy to people living with HIV: the view from Haiti. Antivir Ther. 2014;19(Suppl 3):91-104.

5. The joint United Nations Programme on HIV/AIDS (UNAIDS) data 2019. Public health update. 2020. [Cited 7 July 2020]; Available from: https://www.publichealthupdate.com/the-joint-united-nations-programme-on-hiv-aids-unaids-data-2019.

6. CARICOM. 2016 United Nations political declaration on ending AIDS sets world on the fast-track to end the epidemic by 2030 - CARICOM. CARICOM. 2020. [Cited 7 July 2020]; Available from: https://caricom.org/2016-united-nations-political-declaration-on-ending-aids-sets-world-on-the-fast-track-to-end-the-epidemic-by-2030.

7. Geibel S, Tun W, Tapsoba P, Kellerman S. HIV vulnerability of men who have sex with men in developing countries: horizons studies, 2001–2008. Public Health Rep. 2010;125(2):316-324.

8. Hussen S, Stephenson R, del Rio C, Wilton L, Wallace J, Wheeler D. HIV testing patterns among black men who have sex with men: a qualitative typology. PLoS One. 2013;8(9):e75382.

9. Castro A, Farmer P. Understanding and addressing aids-related stigma: from anthropological theory to clinical practice in Haiti. Am J Public Health. 2005;95(1):53-59.

10. Surkan P, Mukherjee J, Williams D, Eustache E, Louis E, Jean-Paul T, et al. Perceived discrimination and stigma toward children affected by HIV/AIDS and their HIV-positive caregivers in central Haiti. AIDS Care. 2010;22(7):803-815.

11. Abara W, Garba I. HIV epidemic and human rights among men who have sex with men in sub-Saharan Africa: implications for HIV prevention, care, and surveillance. Glob Public Health. 2015;12(4):469-482.

12. Ross M, Nyoni J, Larsson M, Mbwambo J, Agardh A, Kashiha J, et al. Health care in a homophobic climate: the SPEND model for providing sexual health services to men who have sex with men where their health and human rights are compromised. Glob Health Action. 2015;8(1):26096.

13. Beyrer C, Baral S, Collins C, Richardson E, Sullivan P, Sanchez J, et al. The global response to HIV in men who have sex with men. Lancet. 2016;388(10040):198-206.

14. Zukoski A, Thorburn S. Experiences of stigma and discrimination among adults living with HIV in a low HIV-prevalence context: a qualitative analysis. AIDS Patient Care and STDs. 2009;23(4):267-276.

15. Chambers L, Rueda S, Baker D, Wilson M, Deutsch R, Raeifar E, et al. Stigma, HIV and health: a qualitative synthesis. BMC Public Health. 2015;15(1).

16. Walsh K. Attitudes and opinions of medical students concerning HIV and AIDS in Malaysia: the next steps. J Clin Diagnostic Res. 2014;8(10):XL01.

17. Bikmukhametov D, Anokhin V, Vinogradova A, Triner W, McNutt L. Bias in medicine: a survey of medical student attitudes towards HIV-positive and marginalized patients in Russia, 2010. J Int AIDS Soc. 2012; 27;15(2):17372.

18. Matharu K, Kravitz R, McMahon G, Wilson M, Fitzgerald F. Medical students' attitudes toward gay men. BMC Med Educ. 2012;12:71.

19. Alencar Albuquerque G, de Lima Garcia C, da Silva Quirino G, Alves M, Belém J, dos Santos Figueiredo F, et al. Access to health services by lesbian, gay, bisexual, and transgender persons: systematic literature review. BMC Int Health Hum Rights. 2016;16(1).

20. Logie C, Lacombe-Duncan A, Brien N, Jones N, Lee-Foon N, Levermore K et al. Barriers and facilitators to HIV testing among young men who have sex with men and transgender women in Kingston, Jamaica: a qualitative study. J Int AIDS Soc. 2017;20(1):21385.

21. Hall J, Mirza R, Gill P. Leading the way toward a socially-accountable medical education system. Can Med Educ J. 2019;10(1):e128-131.

22. Orisatoki R, Oguntibeju O. Knowledge and attitudes of students in an off-shore Caribbean medical school towards HIV/AIDS. Retrovirology. 2010;7(S1).

23. Sekoni A, Jolly K, Gale N, Ifaniyi O, Somefun E, Agaba E, et al. Provision of healthcare services to men who have sex with men in Nigeria: Students' attitudes following the passage of the same-sex marriage prohibition law. LGBT Health. 2016;3(4):300-307.

24. Programmatic mapping and size estimation of key populations in Haiti. 2017. [Cited 7 July 2020]; Available from: https://www.fhi360.org/sites/default/files/media/documents/resource-linkages-haiti-size-key-populations-april-2017.pdf.

25. Foley G, Timonen V. Using grounded theory method to capture and analyze health care experiences. Health Serv Res. 2014;50(4):1195-1210.

26. Elo S, Kyngäs H. The qualitative content analysis process. J Adv Nurs. 2008;62(1):107-115.

27. Morrow M. Grounded theory. Nurs Sci Q. 2017;30(4):361-361.

28. Cypress B. Rigor or reliability and validity in qualitative research: perspectives, strategies, reconceptualization, and recommendation. Dimens Crit Care Nurs. 2017;36(4):253-263.

29. Korstjens I, Moser A. Series: Practical guidance to qualitative research. Part 4: Trustworthiness and publishing. Eur J Gen Pract. 2017;24(1):120-124.

30. van der Elst E, Smith A, Gichuru E, Wahome E, Musyoki H, Muraguri N, et al. Men who have sex with men sensitivity training reduces homoprejudice and increases knowledge among Kenyan healthcare providers in coastal Kenya. J Int AIDS Soc. 2013;16:18748.

31. Boelen C. Consensus Mondial sur la Responsabilité Sociale des Facultés de Médecine. Santé Publique. 2011;23(3):247.

32. Larkins S, Preston R, Matte M, Lindemann I, Samson R, Tandinco F et al. Measuring social accountability in health professional education: development and international pilot testing of an evaluation framework. Med Teach. 2012;35(1):32-45.

33. Woollard B, Boelen C. Seeking impact of medical schools on health: meeting the challenges of social accountability. Med Educ. 2011;46(1):21-27.

34. Mac-Seing M, Le Nogue D, Bagayoko C, Sy A, Dumas J, Dunbar W, et al. Make visible the invisible: innovative strategies for the future of global health. BMJ Global Health. 2019;4(3):e001693.

35. Muntinga M, Krajenbrink V, Peerdeman S, Croiset G, Verdonk P. Toward diversity-responsive medical education: taking an intersectionality-based approach to a curriculum evaluation. Adv Health Sci Educ Theory Pract. 2015;21(3):541-559.

36. Kapanda L, Jumbe V, Izugbara C, Muula A. Healthcare providers' attitudes towards care for men who have sex with men (MSM) in Malawi. BMC Health Serv Res. 2019;19(1).

37. Matovu J, Musinguzi G, Kiguli J, Nuwaha F, Mujisha G, Musinguzi J, et al. Health providers' experiences, perceptions and readiness to provide HIV services to men who have sex with men and female sex workers in Uganda – a qualitative study. BMC Infect Dis. 2019;19(1).

38. Centers for Disease Control and Prevention. HIV incidence among young men who have sex with men-seven US cities, 1994-2000. JAMA. 2001;286(3):297.

39. Kushwaha S, Lalani Y, Maina G, Ogunbajo A, Wilton L, Agyarko-Poku T, et al. "But the moment they find out that you are MSM…": a qualitative investigation of HIV prevention experiences among men who have sex with men (MSM) in Ghana's health care system. BMC Public Health. 2017;17(1).

40. Rainey S, Trusty J. Attitudes of master's-level counseling students toward gay men and lesbians. Counseling and Values. 2007;52(1):12-24.

41. Hakim A, MacDonald V, Hladik W, Zhao J, Burnett J, Sabin K, et al. Gaps and opportunities: measuring the key population cascade through surveys and services to guide the HIV response. J Int AIDS Soc. 2018;21:e25119.

42. McGrory B, McDowell D, Muskin P. Medical students' attitudes toward AIDS, homosexual, and intravenous drug-abusing patients. Psychosomatics. 1990;31(4):426-433.

43. DeVita T, Bishop C, Plankey M. Queering medical education: systematically assessing LGBTQI health competency and implementing reform. Med Educ Online. 2018;23(1):1510703.

STEP 2 ELICITING MECHANISMS FOR OUTCOMES IMPROVEMENT

To elicit mechanisms for outcomes improvement, two studies were conducted:

The study 4: "A realist systematic review of stigma reduction interventions for HIV prevention and care continuum outcomes among MSM". While stigma associated with HIV infection among men who have sex with men is well recognised, there remains relatively limited intervention data on effective stigma reduction strategies. This systematic review was conducted to highlight the mechanisms through which sexual and HIV stigma is reduced in relation to HIV prevention and care engagement.

The study 5: "A realist evaluation of the continuum of HIV services for men who have sex with men". This evaluation assessed the continuum of HIV services for MSM in Haiti. Guided by a realist approach, an initial program theory (IPT) was developed based on literature and frameworks review, observations and discussions. The IPT was tested using a mixed-method explanatory design. Then, it was refined by eliciting the mechanisms and pathways.

After a description of the contexts from different perspectives, this second step allowed us to elicit the mechanisms through a thoughtful succession of phases as presented in the figure below:

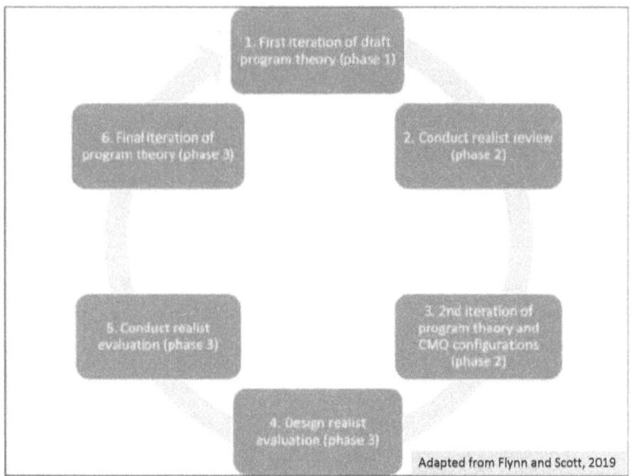

1) First iteration of draft program theory through program framework reviews, discussion with stakeholders and participant observations into the settings and community.

2) Conduct realist review through a systematic literature exploration and analysis leading to the study 4: "A realist systematic review of stigma reduction interventions for HIV prevention and care continuum outcomes among MSM"

3) Second iteration of program theory and CMO configuration resulted from the two previous phases

4) Design realist evaluation from the hypothesis and results of the review

5) Conduct realist evaluation using a mixed method explanatory study: a quantitative phase to build the continuum from a cross-sectional analysis, and a qualitative phase to explore the motivators and facilitators related to proper linkages along the continuum.

6) Final iteration of program theory presenting the motivators and facilitators for the HIV continuum of services through mechanisms and pathways.

Study 4

A realist systematic review of stigma reduction interventions for HIV prevention and care continuum outcomes among men who have sex with men

Willy Dunbar, MD [1] [§], Aline Labat, MPH [1], Nathalie Maulet, PhD [2], Yves Coppieters, MD, PhD [1]

1 Health Systems and Policies - International Health, School of Public Health, Université Libre de Bruxelles (ULB), Brussels, Belgium
2 Institute of Health and Society, Université Catholique de Louvain (UClouvain), Brussels, Belgium

Citation:
Dunbar W, Labat A, Raccurt C, Sohler N, Pape JW, Maulet N, Coppieters Y. A realist systematic review of stigma reduction interventions for HIV prevention and care continuum outcomes among men who have sex with men. Int J STD AIDS. 2020 Jul;31(8):712-723. doi: 10.1177/0956462420924984. PMID: 32631213.

INTERNATIONAL JOURNAL OF
STD &AIDS

International Journal of STD & AIDS
2020, Vol. 31(8) 712–723
© The Author(s) 2020
Article reuse guidelines:
sagepub.com/journals-permissions
DOI: 10.1177/0956462420924984
journals.sagepub.com/home/std

SAGE

A realist systematic review of stigma reduction interventions for HIV prevention and care continuum outcomes among men who have sex with men

Willy Dunbar[1,2], Aline Labat[1], Christian Raccurt[3], Nancy Sohler[4], Jean William Pape[2,5], Nathalie Maulet[6] and Yves Coppieters[1]

Keywords
HIV, stigma, men who have sex with men, systematic review, interventions

Date received: 7 October 2019; accepted: 15 April 2020

Introduction

Since the beginning of the epidemic, human immunodeficiency virus (HIV) has been linked with social stigma.[1] Stigma against people living with HIV (PLHIV), especially sexual minorities, reinforces marginalization and makes access to prevention and care strategies difficult.[2] This has been a significant barrier to effective global response to the epidemic.[3] Despite advances in scientific understanding of HIV, stigmatization continues to be widespread and affect many aspects of life for PLHIV.[4,5]

Goffman distinguished three types of stigma: the first one, physical deformity is a deficit between the

[1]Health Systems and Policies – International Health, School of Public Health, Université Libre de Bruxelles (ULB), Brussels, Belgium
[2]Haitian Study Group for Kaposi's Sarcoma and Opportunistic Infections (GHESKIO), Port-au-Prince, Haiti
[3]Faculty of Health Sciences, Quisqueya University, Port-au-Prince, Haiti
[4]Community Health and Social Medicine, City University of New York, School of Medicine, New York, NY, USA
[5]Center for Global Health, Department of Medicine, Weill Cornell Medical College, New York, NY, USA
[6]Ecole de Santé Publique, Université Catholique de Louvain, Brussels, Belgium

Corresponding author:
Willy Dunbar, École de Santé Publique, Campus Erasme – Bâtiment A, Route de Lennik 808 – CP591, Bruxelles 1070, Belgium.
Email: wdunbar@ulb.ac.be

perfect and the actual physical condition; the second type of stigma is that of character blemishes that may occur in individual with HIV or homosexuality; and the third one, which is prejudice, originates when some features from a group are considered deficient based on another group's socially constructed norm. The second type, character blemishes, is related to this review. PLHIV face considerable stigma because many believe that the infected person could have controlled the behaviours that resulted in the infection.[6,7] In addition, some groups, identities, and behaviours are consistently stigmatized across much of the world. Examples include stigma based on sexual practices and identities of gay men and other men who have sex with men (MSM).[8] From the Joint United Nations Program on HIV/AIDS stigma is also described as a process of devaluation of people either living with or associated with human immunodeficiency virus and acquired immune deficiency syndrome (HIV/AIDS).[9]

MSM, throughout the world, have been one of the constituencies most affected by the HIV pandemic, and continue to be vulnerable to high rates of HIV-related morbidity and mortality relative to other groups.[10-12] The global response to the HIV pandemic has progressed over the decades both in scale and in efforts to reach diverse and vulnerable groups, but stigma and discrimination still follow MSM in many settings.[13] Wanyenze described nine major barriers to HIV treatment and adherence among MSM which can be classified into three groups. The first group is from MSM: fear of being segregated or exposed as MSM, high mobility of the MSM population, and general fears related to HIV-associated stigma and HIV testing. The second group is from the health system: negative attitudes and unwelcoming behaviours of health workers, healthcare workers' lack of sufficient skills and knowledge to manage MSM-specific healthcare needs, limited access to MSM-specific services, and lack of national-level guidelines on how to deal with MSM. The third group is from the community: negative community perceptions towards MSM and harsh legal environment.[14] MSM infected with HIV are subjected to a plethora of unpleasant treatment that includes stigma, discrimination, social ostracism, and violence and continue to be underrepresented in HIV prevention and care programmes.[15]

Despite documented impact of stigma on HIV risks among MSM, there remains relatively limited intervention data on effective stigma reduction interventions for this specific group. While much of the literature has focused on identifying complex causalities that affect HIV incidence among MSM, a few tried to develop and test stigma mitigation interventions to improve HIV prevention and care that address socio-cultural contexts.[16] With this systematic review, we aim to highlight the mechanisms through which stigma mitigation

interventions generate better HIV prevention and contribute to the care continuum for MSM. Our model is developed based on the context in which mechanisms emerge to produce expected outcomes.[17-19] This paper aimed to: (a) review international programme frameworks to develop a preliminary model on stigma reduction interventions for HIV prevention and care outcomes, and (b) refine the preliminary model from a systematic review to identify the mechanisms that have emerged from tested interventions to mitigate stigma and improve HIV outcomes for MSM regarding specific contexts.

Methods

As this work intends to identify mechanisms in complex interventions and different contexts, we used a realist method which is a theory-driven and multi-method-based that uses an interpretive approach to synthesize evidence to reveal how intervention strategies interact with context to trigger mechanisms and produce outcomes. Then, the preliminary programme theory is iteratively refined based on a systematic review of empirical evidence to investigate whether, why, or how intervention strategies produce observed outcomes, for whom and in what circumstances.[18-20]

This work intends to identify mechanisms in complex interventions and different contexts. We used an interpretive approach to synthesize evidence to reveal how intervention strategies interact with context to trigger mechanisms and produce outcomes.[21] Developing effective HIV prevention and treatment strategies requires careful dialogue and greater flexibility for context-specific implementation rather than a one-size-fits-all conceptualization of human rights.[22,23]

In this systematic review, first, we developed a preliminary model to identify how context influences mechanisms to generate outcomes.[20] We conducted a scoping review of the grey literature and international programme frameworks from the United States Agency for International Development (USAID), the U.S. President's Emergency Plan for AIDS Relief (PEPFAR), and the LINKAGES project. Then, the preliminary model is refined based on a systematic review of the literature to investigate whether, why, or how intervention strategies produce observed outcomes, and in what circumstances.

Search strategy and selection criteria

We reviewed the international programme frameworks to develop a preliminary model on stigma reduction interventions for HIV prevention and care outcomes. To test our preliminary model, we performed a systematic search of PubMed and SCOPUS, on March 2019, using MESH terms or other associated terms for HIV cross referenced with 'stigma', 'discrimination reduction', 'social stigma', or 'homophobia', as well as 'men who have sex with men', 'gay men', 'gay man', 'bisexual men', 'bisexual man', 'homosexual men', 'homosexual man', or 'Homosexuality, Male'. Our first screening included studies that described an empirical evaluation of the efficacy or effectiveness of intervention to reduce stigma related to MSM or HIV. Inclusion criteria included presentation of interventions evaluation, clear description of the sampling methods, and stigma mitigation related to MSM or HIV infection as a primary or secondary outcome. Selected qualitative, quantitative, and mixed methods intervention studies from all countries were included. We included ancestry searches of the articles included in the first screening using the same inclusion criteria.

Screening and data abstraction

Two independent reviewers screened each article at the title and abstract (n = 1640) and full-text (n = 140 articles) review stages. All English articles coded as potentially relevant by both reviewers were included for the next stage of the review process. If only one reviewer coded an article as potentially relevant during abstract screening, the review team included that entry for full-text review for increased sensitivity. After full-text review, discrepancies between reviewers regarding inclusion for data abstraction were resolved through discussions until consensus was reached. Finally, 11 studies were included in this review.

Standardized Excel forms were piloted and used for data abstraction. Data were abstracted by two reviewers for each included study using the developed standardized form. The data abstraction form included information about date of data collection, country of study, study aim, intervention strategies, target population, sample size of MSM participants, measured outcomes as defined by the study team (HIV stigma, sexual stigma, or both), what form of stigma was addressed by the intervention, whether/how stigma was measured in the study population, and the underlined structural factors.

There is evidence showing that the interventions described in the studies have been effective in reducing stigma; however, this work shows on how, why, for whom, and in which circumstances particular stigma reduction interventions work. Moreover, there is heterogeneity in the ways in which HIV and sexual stigma is experienced across different communities, and it is likely that the interventions and mechanisms that work to reduce HIV and sexual stigma and improve HIV-related outcomes may also vary between communities and individuals. Thus, this review uses an interpretive approach to synthesize evidence to reveal how intervention strategies interact with context to trigger mechanisms and produce outcomes. The focal point of the analysis was identifying the mechanisms as a basis for constructing the refined model.

Data analysis was conducted qualitatively after extraction. Codes and themes were generated in regard to the context, mechanisms, and intervention strategies. In an iterative way, we followed the process to have the initial model and refine it.

Results

As presented above the preliminary model (Figure 1), we conducted a scoping review of the grey literature and international programme frameworks from the USAID, the PEPFAR, and the LINKAGES project.[24,25] We

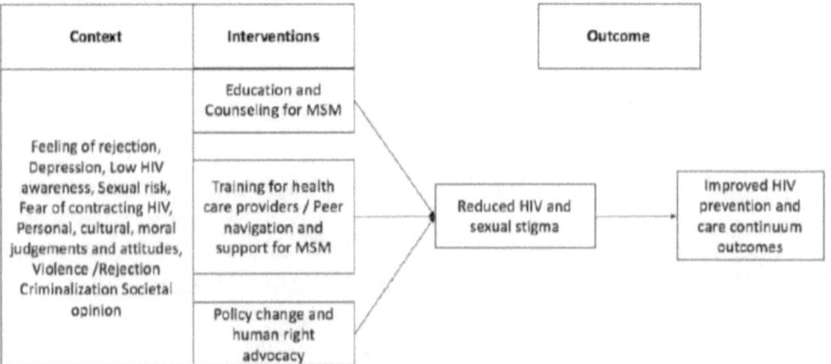

Figure 1. Preliminary model of how stigma reduction interventions improve HIV prevention and care continuum outcomes for MSM. HIV: human immunodeficiency virus; MSM: men who have sex with men.

identified three types of intervention strategies: (1) education and counselling for MSM groups, (2) training for healthcare providers (HCPs) and peer support for linkage and retention to care, and (3) advocacy for policy changes.[26–30] Using these strategies, the goal of interventions is to reduce HIV-related stigma and sexual stigma, and, by doing so improve HIV prevention and care outcomes. Opinions about sexuality and homosexuality are with criminalization part of the structural factors that create and reinforce the stigmatization. Based on such understanding, public messaging, communications, and educational campaigns can be shaped and targeted more effectively for stigma mitigation, resulting in an effective, efficient, equitable, and acceptable HIV response. Interventions including safe spaces for MSM to be educated are very crucial in societies where MSM are victims of ostracism. Given low levels of knowledge observed about risks associated with receptive anal intercourse, providing systematic education about the risks associated with unprotected anal intercourse represents an effective starting point. Supportive policy environments and prioritized HIV prevention programmes for marginalized populations are vital to optimize HIV response.

The initial search strategy identified 2618 entries between the two electronic databases, of which 978 duplicates were removed. Titles and abstracts of the remaining 1640 entries were screened: 1500 were excluded based on eligibility criteria and 140 papers were eligible for full-text review. Of these 140 articles, 129 were excluded and 11 tested interventions manuscripts were included in this review for data abstraction. Out of the 11 selected papers, the proximal outcome was to reduce sexual stigma in five articles, to reduce HIV stigma in two articles, and to reduce HIV and sexual stigma in four articles. However, the distal outcome, which is the main impact of all the studies, was to improve HIV prevention and care continuum outcomes among MSM by reducing HIV and sexual stigma. Our synthesis of all selected articles explained how stigma reduction intervention strategies were implemented in relation to the contextual factors to improve HIV prevention and care continuum outcomes. Among the 11 articles reporting interventions aimed at reducing HIV and sexual stigma in terms of mechanisms, all of them reported improved HIV-related outcomes among MSM. The publication dates

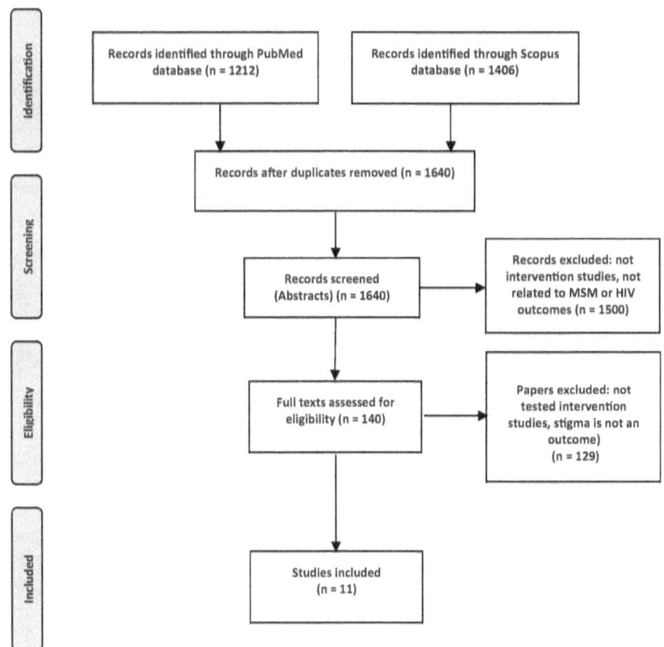

Figure 2. Flow of work processes from the database selection to the screening processes and the final selection of primary studies. HIV: human immunodeficiency virus; MSM: men who have sex with men.

vary from 2013 to 2018. Figure 2 shows the flow of work processes from the database selection to the screening processes and the final selection of primary studies.

Study characteristics

General characteristics and summary of included studies are displayed (Table 1). Seven articles used quantitative methods, two articles used qualitative methods, and two used mixed methods. The countries where the studies were conducted are Bangladesh (1), Kenya (2), Senegal (1), South Africa (2), United States (4), and Thailand (1).

Regarding study samples the populations were MSM only in six studies, MSM and sex workers and HCPs in two studies, HCPs only in two studies, and religious leaders in one study.

Forms of stigma addressed

First, we studied the strategies and analysed them in order to find which form of stigma they addressed. Based on the Valerie Earnshaw[31,32] works,

> People who are HIV infected know that their HIV status is an extremely socially devalued aspect of the self, and this knowledge is experienced through at least three important stigma forms: enacted stigma, anticipated stigma, and internalized stigma. Enacted stigma refers to the degree to which people believe they have actually experienced prejudice and discrimination from others in their community. Anticipated stigma refers to the degree to which people expect that they will experience prejudice and discrimination from others in the future. Internalized stigma refers to the degree to which people endorse the negative beliefs and feelings associated with HIV/AIDS about themselves.

Enacted stigma was decreased by interactive mobile phone- and web-based intervention forum, supportive online community; engagement intervention: training for religious leaders; community intervention (peer-based approach, peer-led session); clinical intervention (training of healthcare workers); and postclinical, web-based referral system intervention (peer-to-peer anonymous referral system); stigma reduction training programme for health service providers; competency training for healthcare workers; self-directed sensitivity training on MSM for healthcare workers. Anticipated stigma was decreased by interactive mobile phone- and web-based intervention forum, supportive online community; educational session programmes. Internalized stigma was decreased by group meetings to facilitate knowledge exchange and disseminate prevention

supplies, intercommunity and community-based activities; interactive mobile phone- and web-based intervention forum, supportive online community; web-based virtual simulation and education; education and peer support; individual motivational-interviewing counselling.

Levels of intervention strategies

Synthesis of all included articles described how stigma reduction interventions were implemented in relation to the contextual factors (Figure 3). The synthesis revealed three different levels of intervention strategies for stigma mitigation, which are explained below. Intrapersonal interventions act on the internalized and anticipated forms of stigma, and interpersonal and structural strategies act on anticipated and enacted forms of stigma. As a result, reduction of HIV and sexual stigma has an impact on HIV prevention and care continuum outcomes which in turn mitigate stigma.

Mechanisms of stigma reduction for HIV prevention and care improvement

Our review found three groups of mechanisms through which HIV and sexual stigma can be reduced in MSM populations. These mechanisms were determined by the components of the interventions and the specific contexts. We present the mechanisms and for each of them the strategies through which they were identified.

Mechanism 1: Self-acceptance, leadership, and motivational activation for behaviour change

This mechanism is a trajectory using hope and confidence to achieve a complete acceptation of HIV status and sexual orientation. Different motivation may be linked to an activation of a series of positive actions that lead to behaviour change. From intrapersonal strategies, such as education and mobile health strategies, which intervene on internalized and anticipated stigma self-acceptance, leadership and motivational activation for behaviour change are identified.

Intrapersonal intervention strategies

Education for MSM. As part of the intrapersonal strategies, education for MSM represented a key strategy for stigma reduction. Education provides opportunities both to learn about sexuality and to express feeling through social activities. To illustrate, one education method adopted a family structure that also serves as a refuge for MSM while providing social support and guidance. With a decline in stigma, participants were empowered to use their natural leadership skills to influence their friends and acquaintances to protect themselves from HIV.[33]

able 1. Summary of included studies.

thor	Country	Study design	Study aims	Intervention target groups	MSM sample size	Strategies	Interventions	Forms of stigma addressed	Measured outcomes	Impacts	Stigma measurement methods	Related contextual factors	Results
:ist et al.[37]	South Africa	Qualitative	To disseminate and promote HIV prevention information, supplies, and service uptake	MSM	98	Intrapersonal and interpersonal	Group meetings to facilitate knowledge exchange and disseminate prevention supplies, intercommunity and community-based activities	Perceived and internalized	Sexual stigma	HIV prevention outcomes	Qualitatively	Community and individual	Participants reported gaining access to MSM-specific HIV prevention information. Improvement of feelings of loneliness, social isolation, self-esteem and self-efficacy.
,ermeister et al.[35]	United States	Mixed methods	To evaluate sexual and HIV stigma, to explore and examine whether changes in stigma occur over time	MSM	238	Intrapersonal	Interactive mobile phone- and web-based intervention forum/supportive online community	Enacted, perceived, anticipated, and internalized	HIV and sexual stigma	HIV prevention and care continuum outcomes	Stewart's 10-item subscale on felt-normative stigma; questions focused on perceptions regarding LGBTQ prejudice; 5-item internalized homophobia scale	Individual	Participants who challenged sexuality-related stigma in forums had lower internalized homophobia at baseline.
ristensen et al.[34]	United States	Quantitative	To test the effectiveness of Socially Optimized Learning in Virtual Environments (SOLVE) in reducing shame	MSM	935	Intrapersonal	Web-based virtual simulation and education	Internalized	Sexual stigma	HIV prevention outcomes	Scale from Watson and Clark's (1994)[44-46]	Individual	At baseline, MSM reporting more risky sexual behaviour reported more shame. MSM in the intervention reported more shame reduction which in turn predicted reductions in risky sexual behaviour at follow-up.
:huru et al.[43]	Kenya	Qualitative	To describe and test the implementation of an engagement intervention towards the reduction of stigmatization and increased social acceptance of GBMSM with religious leaders	Religious leaders	N/A	Structural	Engagement intervention: training for religious leaders	Enacted	HIV and sexual stigma	HIV prevention and care continuum outcomes	Qualitatively	Structural	Many religious leaders, who initially expressed exceedingly negative attitudes towards MSM, started to express far more accepting and supportive views of sexuality, sexual identities, and same-sex relations.
.sek et al.[33]	United States	Quantitative	To evaluate feasibility, acceptability, and preliminary efficacy of an evidence-based, community-level popular opinion leader (OL) intervention	MSM	406	Intrapersonal and interpersonal	Education and peer support	Perceived and internalized	HIV stigma	HIV prevention outcomes	HIV Stigma Scale[45]	Individual and community	Declines were observed for multiple sexual partners, condomless anal intercourse, and HIV stigma.
,ns et al.[39]	Senegal	Quantitative	To evaluate the impact of the three-tiered integrated stigma mitigation interventions (ISMIs) approach to optimizing HIV service delivery for key populations in Senegal	MSM and FSW	724	Intrapersonal, interpersonal, and health systems-related	Community intervention (peer-based approach, peer-led session); clinical intervention (training of healthcare workers); and post-clinical, web-based referral system intervention (peer-to-peer anonymous referral system).	Enacted and perceived	Sexual stigma	HIV prevention and care continuum outcomes	Contextual questions at baseline, three-month and six-month assessments	Health system, community, individual	Overall, 63.9% of MSM agreed that the intervention is effective in addressing stigma; baseline data reinforce the need for stigma mitigation interventions, combined with enhanced linkage and retention to optimize HIV treatment.

103

(continued)

able 1. Continued

thor	Country	Study design	Study aims	Intervention target groups	MSM sample size	Strategies	Interventions	Forms of stigma addressed	Measured outcomes	Impacts	Stigma measurement methods	Related contextual factors	Results
lendez et al.[38]	United States	Mixed Methods	To conduct and evaluate a pilot HIV prevention intervention that asks men to discuss and explore issues relating to their families and sexual disclosures	MSM	44	Intrapersonal and interpersonal	12-session programme offered over a six-week period guided by Paulo Freire's principle of 'popular education'	Internalized and anticipated	Sexual stigma	HIV prevention outcomes	Qualitatively	Individual and community	Survey results indicate that after their participation in the programme, partici-pants increased their safer sex behaviours, comfort disclosing their sexual orientation and support from friends.
ngkavilit et al.[36]	Thailand	Quantitative	To present a further analysis of the effect of Healthy Choices among HIV+ young Thai MSM population	MSM	74	Intrapersonal	Individual motivational-interviewing counselling	Internalized and perceived	HIV stigma	HIV care continu-um outcomes (adherence)	Berger's 40-item HIV Stigma Scale[45]	Individual and community	Improvements in mental health and HIV stigma were noted in Intervention group. Healthy Choices is a promising behavioural intervention and should be further developed.
ibel et al.[41]	Bangladesh	Quantitative	To assess the effects of the stigma reduction trainings on service provider atti-tudes, as well as young client satisfaction with services	HCP, MSM, and sex workers	94	Interpersonal and health systems related	Stigma reduction train-ing programme for health service providers	Enacted and perceived	HIV and sexual stigma	HIV prevention and care continuum outcomes	With a series of ques-tions to assess per-sonal drivers of stigma and discrimination	Health system, individual	Provider agreement that sex-ually active men who have sex with men engage in 'immoral behavior' decreased substantially.
:ker et al.[42]	South Africa	Quantitative	To evaluate the efficacy of MSM Competency Training for healthcare workers administered by Health4Men	HCP	N/A	Health systems-related	Competency training for healthcare workers	Enacted	Sexual stigma	HIV prevention and care continuum outcomes	With questions regard-ing 'sensitivity' knowledge; 25 ques-tion Likert scale on homoprejudicial attitudes	Health system	After training, both clinicians and clinic support staff showed an increase in knowledge and a reduc-tion in homoprejudicial attitude scores.
ı der Elst EM et al.[40]	Kenya	Quantitative	To assess the feasibility of a web-based, self-directed learning of MSM health issues and evaluate the effect of the training intervention upon HCW knowledge and attitudes	HCP	N/A	Health systems-related	Self-directed sensitivity training on MSM for healthcare workers	Enacted	HIV and sexual stigma	HIV prevention and care continuum outcomes	Homophobic scale (HS)[46]	Health system	Compared to baseline, homophobic attitudes had decreased significantly three months after train-ing, particularly among HCW with high homo-phobia scores at baseline, and there was some evi-dence of correlation between improvements in knowledge and reduction in homophobic sentiment.

W: female sex worker; HCP: healthcare provider; HCW: health care workers; HIV: human immunodeficiency virus; MSM: men who have sex with men.

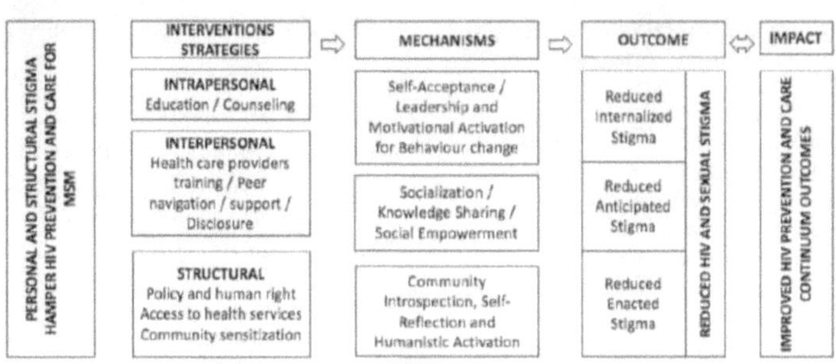

Figure 3. Refined model illustrating the mechanisms through which the intervention strategies reduce stigma and improve HIV prevention and care continuum improvement. HIV: human immunodeficiency virus; MSM: men who have sex with men.

Mobile and online health interventions. Online strategies to reduce stigma have two components: addressing feelings of shame and increasing interactive discussion. Strategies that act against shame are associated with sexual stigma by enabling MSM to more consciously acknowledge their desires and to recognize that their desires are normal. With sexual shame reduction, rates of unprotected anal sex were also indirectly decreased. These findings suggested that, for some MSM, shame reduction may be an important intervention component resulting in HIV prevention and care enrolment.[34] There were online forums and message boards to understand MSM's perceptions, attitudes, and experiences regarding sexual and HIV-related content. Accessible from any location convenient to the participant, it promoted interactive discussions between peers. MSM were empowered, less stigmatized, and were educated about sexuality and HIV.[35]

Individual motivational-interviewing (MI) counselling. This strategy was previously tested and worked in the United States then it was conducted in Thailand through a randomized trial with a four-session MI intervention that lasts 1–1.5 h. The sessions in both groups occurred at 1, 2, 6, and 12 weeks after the baseline visit. Associated with sexual risk reduction and improvement in HIV stigma, MI counselling is a collaborative, client-centred counselling style designed to increase motivational readiness to behaviour change by exploring ambivalence about change, eliciting discrepancies between current behaviours and personal goals, and building self-efficacy.[36]

Mechanism 2: Socialization, knowledge sharing, and social empowerment

Socialization with peers where MSM can share their experience and knowledge not only gives them a chance to learn from each other but also to express their expertise about the adequate way they should be treated through a participatory approach. This mechanism shows how they may be retained in the healthcare continuum through solid patient–caregiver relationships. From interpersonal strategies, such as peer support and training for care providers' socialization, knowledge sharing and social empowerment are developed.

Interpersonal intervention strategies

Support group meetings. The first study about support group meetings was conducted in South Africa where group meetings took place every 1–2 weeks, were semi-structured, and included both social and educational components. Support group meetings promoted knowledge sharing and socializing between MSM. With indoor and outdoor activities this strategy promoted knowledge sharing, socializing between MSM, and helped them to better prepare for and mitigate the effects of stigma and prejudice.[37]

Another form of support group meeting was a 12-session programme offered over a six-week period in the USA to address issues of disclosure of sexual orientation, family rejection, and issues relating to oppression for MSM. Discussion allowed for cultural nuances to shine through from the participants. Survey results indicate that after their participation in the programme, participants increased their safer sex behaviours, comfort disclosing their sexual orientation and support from friends. The implication is that HIV prevention needs to incorporate cultural, social, and structural factors.[38]

Community-based activities.
With several modules, the community interventions aimed to cover topics like HIV prevention and transmission; human rights; stigma and discrimination; reproductive health; and living with HIV. Topics included HIV transmission and prevention, and risk reduction techniques; definitions of human rights and rights issues in the MSM community; and methods for identifying and responding to stigma and discrimination, stress management, and self-esteem. Additional topics included sexual health, nutrition specific information for PLHIV, disease progression, well-being, and life balance. The intervention was delivered by peer educators and all modules were adapted to reflect MSM specific needs.[37,39]

Health-based interventions.

- Peer support:
  This intervention operationalized a referral system designed to provide users anonymous and real-time feedback and recommendations for where friendly, non-stigmatizing health services may be accessed. This intervention aimed to provide an anonymous reference system for health services and prevention information between peers of the cohort participants.[39]

- Training for HCPs: Some studies assessed the effectiveness of several training interventions for the HCPs. They aimed at addressing enacted stigma and alleviating barriers to care for MSM on the part of the HCPs. It improved the clinical and social competency of the providers in addressing the needs of MSM. Topics included sex, sexuality, and sexual health; mental health promotion; overcoming barriers; creating a friendlier environment; health implications of sexual practices; assessing health status; evidence-based interventions; clinical care for HIV and other sexually transmitted infections; gender-based violence; and reproductive health.[39,40] After the interventions, fear-based and value-based stigma were significantly reduced. The participatory stigma training methods utilized here can be a valuable tool to help providers reflect on their own values, attitudes, and practices.[41] The results also supported claims that a lack of knowledge regarding a stigmatized group was often associated with negative attitudes about that group,

while also elaborating on potential complexities in this relationship.[37,42]

Mechanism 3: Community introspection, self-reflection, and humanistic activation

Engagement, collaboration, and reflection exercises are used to help community members becoming aware of their own stigmatizing actions so they can transform their habitual use of discriminatory language and action. For this case, religious leaders showed the ability to gradually apply more humanistic, caring discourse towards MSM indicating attitude's change and socialization. From structural mechanisms, such as community leaders' sensitization, which both intervene on anticipated and enacted stigma community introspection, self-reflection and humanistic activation are reached.

Structural intervention strategies

Training for religious leaders. One study showed positive results after working with religious leaders in HIV prevention. Workshops were held with them and addressed the following topics: MSM and HIV; stigma; identity, coming out, and disclosure; anal sex and common sexual practices; HIV and sexually transmitted infections; mental health, anxiety, depression, and substance abuse; HIV prevention measures; and risk reduction counselling. Approaches for reducing stigma generated introspection and self-reflection. Religious leaders also showed that they were able to gradually apply more humanistic, caring discourse, indicating that one can interrupt the cycle of socialization and stand up for change.[43]

Discussion

Evidence indicates that stigma meets all of the criteria to be considered as a fundamental barrier for prevention and treatment of HIV in MSM populations. Based on their sexuality, behaviour, and their HIV status, MSM confront multiple layers of stigmatization and discrimination. Even though research on intervention against stigma has increased throughout the evolution of HIV disease, more activities are required to fully assess the extent, consequences, and potential countermeasures in relation to HIV-related stigma within MSM communities.[4] Despite many descriptive and intervention studies, HIV stigma continues to hamper prevention and treatment strategies.[31]

The findings from this review helped us highlight the mechanisms through which stigma can be mitigated. Self-acceptance, leadership, and motivational activation for behaviour change is a key component to intrapersonal strategies. MSM felt more confident and this mechanism is built by sharing a focus on greater self-awareness of emotions, goals, behaviours, and associated barriers while fostering acceptance of parts of the self that cannot change. Socialization, knowledge sharing, and social empowerment allow MSM to help their peers not only for stigma reduction but also for engagement and retention in care. Training sessions for care givers allow them to better understand the specificities of MSM and allow them to have appropriate knowledge. Community introspection, self-reflection, and humanistic activation allow structural changes through community engagement.

There were 11 evaluated interventions with focus on reducing stigma in MSM communities. These interventions have been shown to be effective, but have been tested in different countries with sample size variation from 44 MSM to 935 MSM and over periods that vary from several weeks to months. Many gaps remain, especially in relation to the impact of these strategies, the sample size, the duration of the interventions, and the transferability in terms of contextual differences. The impact of stigma spreads throughout MSM's lives causing home loss, school dropout, instability in the job market, and limited willingness and ability to seek care. This means economic and physical factors that contribute to loss to follow-up. Other factors involved in loss to follow-up, including economic and physical factors, need to be addressed to optimize HIV outcomes. Combination of larger structural interventions like large scale public campaigns, awareness, and education in schools and specific communities and civil society movements with personal interventions is essential to encouraging societies to embrace diversity.

Several intervention strategies, such as the training for HCPs and religious leaders, show how specific training sessions lead to changes in stigmatizing attitudes and behaviours against MSM. These strategies, however, do not sufficiently consider intrapersonal mechanisms of stigma generation. It appears that stigma interventions are more effective when multiple strategies are implemented together to address complex health programmes, such as the HIV prevention and care continuum. Our model provides sufficient evidence to claim that multi-level intervention strategies are essential for stigma mitigation.

Refining the initial model, we found that some interventions considered that all MSM lack knowledge on HIV services, but in other studies MSM are viewed as experts in their lives and challenges to safer sex behaviour. Sharing sessions rather than formal training can also be one of the components of programmes. This approach allows for various contextual nuances to shine through from the MSM rather than the experts.

This review was limited since it did not include all the available literature on interventions for MSM since there was a focus on the ones that were tested. So, we may have missed some aspects of the socio-cultural contexts and mechanisms. Another limitation is the subjective aspect of qualitative form of analysis and data interpretation through the process even if discussions to reach consensus were central among the team. Because of that, we were not specific in defining which particular interventions or the components of the intervention were more effective.

Despite these limitations, the review also was based on the psychological mechanisms of stigma and tried to develop a model that considered all the components. Besides, the scope of the review included papers from a global perspective which was not limited to one region. We believe that the multiple contexts lying behind the interventions added value in trying to reach a saturation point in refining the preliminary model. Thus, we propose that the model outlined in this review should be seen as a contribution to stigma reduction and HIV prevention and care for MSM. As a realist review seeks not to judge but to explain, and is driven by the question 'What works for whom in what circumstances and in what respects' we found that the intervention mechanisms in the refined programme theory act complementarily and can be adapted in terms of different socio-structural and cultural contexts in which MSM exposed to and infected with HIV are living.

Authors' contributions

WD, AL, NS, CR, JWP, and YC conceived the original research idea and led the design of the study. WD, AL, and NS conducted the screening of the papers. WD, AL, and NS conducted the data extraction and WD and NS conducted the analysis. WD, AL, NS, CR, JWP, NM, and YC provided insights in the final programme theory. WD developed the first draft of the article. WD, AL, NS, NM, and YC oversaw the development and revision of the article and contributed to the revisions. All authors reviewed and approved the final draft.

Acknowledgements

Authors would like to acknowledge Valérie Durieux from the Bibliothèque des Sciences de la Santé, Université libre de Bruxelles (ULB), Belgium for her help and support during the study.

Declaration of conflicting interests

Funding

The authors received no financial support for the research, authorship, and/or publication of this article.

ORCID iD

Willy Dunbar https://orcid.org/0000-0002-9134-9288

References

1. Berg RC and Ross MW. The second closet: a qualitative study of HIV stigma among seropositive gay men in a southern U.S. city. *Int J Sex Health* 2014; 26: 186–199.
2. Lebouché B and Et Lévy JJ. Récits de souffrance et VIH/sida: réflexions sur quelques enjeux anthropologiques et éthiques du témoignage . *Alterstice* 2011; 1: 98–107.
3. Mahajan AP, Sayles JN, Patel VA, et al. Stigma in the HIV/AIDS epidemic: a review of the literature and recommendations for the way forward. *AIDS* 2008; 22: S67–S79.
4. Smit PJ, Brady M, Carter M, et al. HIV-related stigma within communities of gay men: a literature review. *AIDS Care* 2012; 24: 405–412.
5. Stangl AL, Earnshaw VA, Logie CH, et al. The health stigma and discrimination framework: a global, crosscutting framework to inform research, intervention development, and policy on health-related stigmas. *BMC Med* 2019; 17: 31.
6. Wiener C (ed.) and Srauss A (ed.). *Where medicine fails.* New York: Routledge, 1997.
7. Goffman E. *Stigmate, les usages sociaux des handicaps.* Paris: Les Éditions de Minuit, 1975.
8. Fitzgerald-Husek A, Van Wert MJ, Ewing WF, et al. Measuring stigma affecting sex workers (SW) and men who have sex with men (MSM): a systematic review. *PLoS One* 2017; 12: e0188393.
9. Joint United Nations Program on HIV/AIDS. Stigma and discrimination: facts sheet on HIV/AIDS, 2003.
10. Amirkhanian YA. Social networks, sexual networks and HIV risk in men who have sex with men. *Curr HIV/AIDS Rep* 2014; 11: 81–92.
11. Cáceres CF. HIV among gay and other men who have sex with men in Latin America and the Caribbean: a hidden epidemic? *AIDS* 2002; 16: S23–S33.
12. Papworth E, Ceesay N, An L, et al. Epidemiology of HIV among female sex workers, their clients, men who have sex with men and people who inject drugs in West and Central Africa. *J Int AIDS Soc* 2013; 16: 18751.
13. Goffman E. *Stigma: notes on the management of spoiled identity.* Englewood Cliffs, NJ: Prentice-Hall, 1963.
14. Wanyenze RK, Musinguzi G, Matovu JK, et al. "If you tell people that you had sex with a fellow man, it is hard to be helped and treated": barriers and opportunities for increasing access to HIV services among men who have sex with men in Uganda. *PLoS One* 2016; 11: e0147714.
15. Baral S, Sifakis F, Cleghorn F, et al. Elevated risk for HIV infection among men who have sex with men in low- and middle-income countries 2000–2006: a systematic review. *PLoS Med* 2007; 4: e339.
16. Hightow-Weidman L, LeGrand S, Choi SK, et al. Exploring the HIV continuum of care among young black MSM. *PLoS One* 2017; 12: e0179688.
17. Pawson R, Greenhalgh T, Harvey G, et al. Realist review – a new method of systematic review designed for complex policy interventions. *J Health Serv Res Policy* 2005; 10: 21–34.
18. Pawson R. Evidence-based policy: a realist perspective. In: Carter B and New C (eds) *Making realism work: realist social theory and empirical research.* London: Routledge, 2004, pp. 26–49.
19. Pawson R and Tilley N. Realistic evaluation bloodlines. *Am J Eval* 2001; 22: 317–324.
20. Triana R. Evidence-based policy: a realist perspective, by Ray Pawson. *J Policy Pract* 2008; 7: 321–323.
21. de Souza DE. Elaborating the context-mechanism-outcome configuration (CMOc) in realist evaluation: a critical realist perspective. *Evaluation* 2013; 19: 141–154.
22. Muzyamba C, Broaddus E and Campbell C. "You cannot eat rights": a qualitative study of views by Zambian HIV-vulnerable women, youth and MSM on human rights as public health tools. *BMC Int Health Hum Rights* 2015; 15: 26.
23. Amon JJ and Kasambala T. Structural barriers and human rights related to HIV prevention and treatment in Zimbabwe. *Glob Public Health* 2009; 4: 528–545.
24. Mills S and Francis C. HIV cascade framework for key populations. Linkages, http://data.unaids.org/publications/fact-sheets03/fs_stigma_discrimination_en.pdf (2015, accessed 7 October 2019).
25. Needle R, Fu J, Beyrer C, et al. PEPFAR's evolving HIV prevention approaches for key populations–people who inject drugs, men who have sex with men, and sex workers: progress, challenges, and opportunities. *J Acquir Immune Defic Syndr* 2012; 60: S145–S151.
26. van der Elst EM, Kombo B, Gichuru E, et al. The green shoots of a novel training programme: progress and identified key actions to providing services to MSM at Kenyan health facilities. *J Int AIDS Soc* 2015; 18: 20226.
27. Wirtz AL, Trapence G, Jumbe V, et al. Feasibility of a combination HIV prevention program for men who have sex with men in Blantyre, Malawi. *J Acquir Immune Defic Syndr* 2015; 70: 155–162.
28. Ross MW, Nyoni J, Larsson M, et al. Health care in a homophobic climate: the SPEND model for providing sexual health services to men who have sex with men where their health and human rights are compromised. *Glob Health Action* 2015; 8: 26096.
29. Graham SM, Micheni M, Kombo B, et al. Development and pilot testing of an intervention to promote care engagement and adherence among HIV-positive Kenyan MSM. *AIDS* 2015; 29: S241–S249.
30. Tucker A, de Swardt G, Struthers H, et al. Understanding the needs of township men who have sex with men (MSM) health outreach workers: exploring the interplay between volunteer training, social capital and critical consciousness. *AIDS Behav* 2013; 17: S33–S42.

31. Earnshaw VA and Chaudoir SR. From conceptualizing to measuring HIV stigma: a review of HIV stigma mechanism measures. *AIDS Behav* 2009; 13: 1160–1177.
32. Earnshaw VA, Smith LR, Chaudoir SR, et al. HIV stigma mechanisms and well-being among PLWH: a test of the HIV stigma framework. *AIDS Behav* 2013; 17: 1785–1795.
33. Hosek SG, Lemos D, Hotton AL, et al. An HIV intervention tailored for black young men who have sex with men in the House Ball Community. *AIDS Care* 2015; 27: 355–362.
34. Christensen JL, Miller LC, Appleby PR, et al. Reducing shame in a game that predicts HIV risk reduction for young adult MSM: a randomized trial delivered nationally over the Web. *J Int AIDS Soc* 2013; 16: 18716.
35. Bauermeister JA, Muessig KE, LeGrand S, et al. HIV and sexuality stigma reduction through engagement in online forums: results from the HealthMPowerment intervention. *AIDS Behav* 2019; 23: 742–752.
36. Rongkavilit C, Wang B, Naar-King S, et al. Motivational interviewing targeting risky sex in HIV-positive young Thai men who have sex with men. *Arch Sex Behav* 2015; 44: 329–340.
37. Batist E, Brown B, Scheibe A, et al. Outcomes of a community-based HIV-prevention pilot programme for township men who have sex with men in Cape Town, South Africa. *J Int AIDS Soc* 2013; 16: 18754.
38. Melendez RM, Zepeda J, Samaniego R, et al. "La Familia" HIV prevention program: a focus on disclosure and family acceptance for Latino immigrant MSM to the USA. *Salud Publica Mex* 2013; 55: S491–S497.
39. Lyons CE, Ketende S, Diouf D, et al. Potential impact of integrated stigma mitigation interventions in improving HIV/AIDS service delivery and uptake for key populations in Senegal. *J Acquir Immune Defic Syndr* 2017; 74: S52–S59.
40. van der Elst EM, Smith AD, Gichuru E, et al. Men who have sex with men sensitivity training reduces homoprejudice and increases knowledge among Kenyan healthcare providers in coastal Kenya. *J Int AIDS Soc* 2013; 16: 18748.
41. Geibel S, Hossain SM, Pulerwitz J, et al. Stigma reduction training improves healthcare provider attitudes toward, and experiences of, young marginalized people in Bangladesh. *J Adolesc Health* 2017; 60: S35–S44.
42. Tucker A, Liht J, de Swardt G, et al. Efficacy of tailored clinic trainings to improve knowledge of men who have sex with men health needs and reduce homoprejudicial attitudes in South Africa. *LGBT Health* 2016; 3: 443–450.
43. Gichuru E, Kombo B, Mumba N, et al. Engaging religious leaders to support HIV prevention and care for gays, bisexual men, and other men who have sex with men in coastal Kenya. *Crit Public Health* 2018; 28: 294–305.
44. Watson D and Clark LA. Introduction to the special issue on personality and psychopathology. *J Abnormal Psych* 1994; 103: 3–5.
45. Berger BE, Ferrans CE and Lashley FR. Measuring stigma in people with HIV: psychometric assessment of the HIV stigma scale. *Res Nurs Health* 2001; 24: 518–529.
46. Wright LW, Adams HE and Bernat J. Development and Validation of the Homophobia Scale. *J Psychopath and Behav Assess* 1999; 21: 337–347.

Presentation of the study 5:

The realist review synthesized the evidences of stigma reduction interventions by an interpretative theory-driven approach using. We developed a preliminary model to identify how context influences mechanisms to generate outcomes. We conducted a scoping review of the grey literature and international program frameworks from the United States Agency for International Development (USAID), the U.S. President's Emergency Plan for AIDS Relief (PEPFAR) and the LINKAGES project. Then, the preliminary model was refined based on a systematic review of the literature to investigate whether, why, or how intervention strategies produce observed outcomes, and in what circumstances.

The results led to the design and conduct of the realist evaluation by a second and a final iteration of the program theory and CMO configuration to elicit the mechanisms and pathways for an overall improved continuum of HIV services.

Study 5

A realist evaluation of the continuum of HIV services for men who have sex with men

Willy Dunbar, MD [1][§], Aline Labat, MPH [1], Nathalie Maulet, PhD [2], Yves Coppieters, MD, PhD [1]

1 Health Systems and Policies - International Health, School of Public Health, Université Libre de Bruxelles (ULB), Brussels, Belgium
2 Institute of Health and Society, Université Catholique de Louvain (UClouvain), Brussels, Belgium

A realist evaluation of the continuum of HIV services for men who have sex with men

Willy Dunbar, MD [1][§], Aline Labat, MPH [1], Nathalie Maulet, PhD [2], Yves Coppieters, MD, PhD [1]

1 Health Systems and Policies - International Health, School of Public Health, Université Libre de Bruxelles (ULB), Brussels, Belgium
2 Institute of Health and Society, Université Catholique de Louvain (UClouvain), Brussels, Belgium

[§] Corresponding author: Willy Dunbar

A realist evaluation of the continuum of HIV services for men who have sex with men

Abstract

Introduction:

Men who have Sex with Men (MSM) represent the risk group that are disproportionately most affected by human immunodeficiency virus (HIV), yet are understudied in intervention research. This realist evaluation assessed the continuum of HIV services for MSM in Haiti.

Methods:

Guided by a realist approach, an initial program theory (IPT) was developed based on literature and frameworks review, observations and discussions. The IPT was tested using a mixed-method explanatory study. Then, it was refined by eliciting the mechanisms and pathways.

Results:

The results showed that the current service delivery model is suboptimal in engaging and retaining MSM, resulting in loss to follow-up at every step of the continuum and failure to fully realize the health and prevention benefits of antiretroviral. However, the mechanisms through which linkages across the continuum can be improved are: self-acceptance, sense of community support and sense of comprehensive and tailored HIV services.

Conclusion:

The continuum of HIV services for MSM is affected by a multi-layer of factors, thus highlighting the importance of taking a comprehensive approach to improve the program.

Keywords: HIV; Men who have Sex with Men; Stigma; Context-Mechanism-Outcome configuration; Care continuum; Realist evaluation.

A realist evaluation of the continuum of HIV services for men who have sex with men

Introduction

Men who have sex with men (MSM) represent the risk group that are disproportionately affected by the human immunodeficiency virus (HIV) compared to the general population (1). Data suggest that the risk of HIV acquisition among MSM was 22 times higher than it was among all adult men in 2018(2). Despite progress to control the HIV among MSM, biological, behavioral, legal, socio-cultural factors continue to hamper the global response (3). Around the world — even in countries where same-sex practices, relationships, and marriages are legal — discrimination and homophobia persist. In varying degrees, this can impact MSM's ability and willingness to access high-quality health services and information (4). In many settings, criminalization of consensual, adult same-sex behavior, stigma, discrimination and violence against MSM has created an environment which compromises people's human rights and where they are less likely to access essential health and HIV services (5).

As the health and prevention benefits of antiretroviral therapy (ART) in the management of HIV are now well documented, the world is currently pushing for fast-track in driving the 95–95–95 targets: that by 2030, 95% of people living with HIV know their HIV status, 95% of people who know their status are receiving treatment and 95% of people on HIV treatment have a suppressed viral load (6). Behavioral prevention programs, early diagnosis, prompt linkage to sustained care, retention in care, receipt of ART, and viral suppression constitute points along a comprehensive continuum of HIV services. The term continuum refers to this sequence of steps a person with HIV takes from diagnosis, through linkage to care, receiving treatment until viral load is suppressed to undetectable levels. Each step in the continuum is marked by an assessment of the number of people who have reached that stage (7,8). However, current service delivery models are less than optimal in referring, linking and retaining MSM, resulting in lost to follow-up (LTFU) in the continuum of care and failure to fully realize the benefits of ART (9,10).

In Haiti, although the response to HIV has seen important advances and continued reduction in incidence and expansion of treatment access for those living with HIV, the epidemic in MSM remains severe and yet poorly studied (11). This is clearly one of the defining challenges ahead in the effort to control the HIV in the country. The past years has seen notable progress with a declining HIV prevalence, and treatment outcomes. This success is tied to a strong foundation for HIV care that has contributed in reducing the national HIV prevalence from 6.2% in 1993 to 2.0 % in 2018 (11,12). However, the HIV prevalence among MSM was 18.2% in 2017 making them the most underserved population in term of HIV prevention and care. MSM are not yet adequately represented in the literature on HIV and of particular concern is the lack of data on the continuum of HIV services in Haiti, which is necessary to measure national progress against UNAIDS 95-95-95 targets (6,13). In addition, research methodologies that account for the role that contextual factors play - instead of controlling them - have still been scarcely used to improve the HIV services uptake among MSM (14).

As various strategies have been adopted to overcome some of the challenges cited above, the Linkages Across the Continuum of HIV Services for Key Populations Affected by HIV (LINKAGES) Program has been developed. Evaluations to assess the level of implementation of this intervention targeted MSM along the continuum are needed. Most importantly, studies to highlight the mechanisms that trigger linkage and retention in care are important. This article aims to fill this knowledge gap by: 1) describing the evaluation carried out in Haiti aiming to ascertain why, how and under which circumstances MSM are linked and retained along the care continuum, 2) assessing the outcomes of this approach and 3) exploring the motivators and facilitators for the HIV continuum of services through mechanisms and pathways. .

Methods

Study conceptual framework

In this study, we applied the realist evaluation approach to explore the linkages across the continuum of HIV services for MSM in Haiti. Realist evaluation, proven to be useful when exploring complex health systems interventions, asks 'what works?', and also 'how or why does this work, for whom, in what circumstances?' (15). The nature of realist evaluation lies in its conceptualization of the context, the mechanism and the outcome of a complex intervention (16,17). It starts by eliciting an initial program theory (IPT) which is tested through research. The data analysis serves to refine the IPT while identifying the mechanisms that trigger linkages and retention (18,19).

Overview of the LINKAGES

The LINKAGES is a project that aims to accelerate the ability of governments, MSM organizations and private sector providers to collaboratively plan, deliver and optimize services that reduce HIV transmission among MSM and extend life for those who are HIV-positive. This intervention works with multiple stakeholders by: 1) identifying MSM and comprehensively assessing risk and service access, 2) diagnosing "leaks" within the HIV services cascade, 3) scaling up "what works" while innovating to ensure the most strategic use of resources and access to newly emerging technologies, 4) pulling down structural barriers and transforming MSM organizations, and 5) ensuring MSM interventions are sustainable (4). The approach is summarized in the cascade framework that presents services along a continuum of HIV prevention, diagnosis, care, treatment, and viral suppression (Figure 1). The cascade is aligned with the United Nations 95–95–95 targets.

We conducted the present study at the Groupe Haitien d'Etude du Sarcome de Kaposi et des Infections Opportunistes (GHESKIO) in Port-au-Prince, Haïti. GHESKIO works with the Haitian Government to implement the prevention and care model to a network of 27 healthcare centers throughout the country through training, monitoring and evaluation. This seamless integration of intervention components requires strong linkages among program elements so that HIV transmission is reduced and MSM diagnosed with HIV obtain early access to services. Thus, this model necessitates that MSM flow efficiently, consistently, and sustainably through the entire continuum.

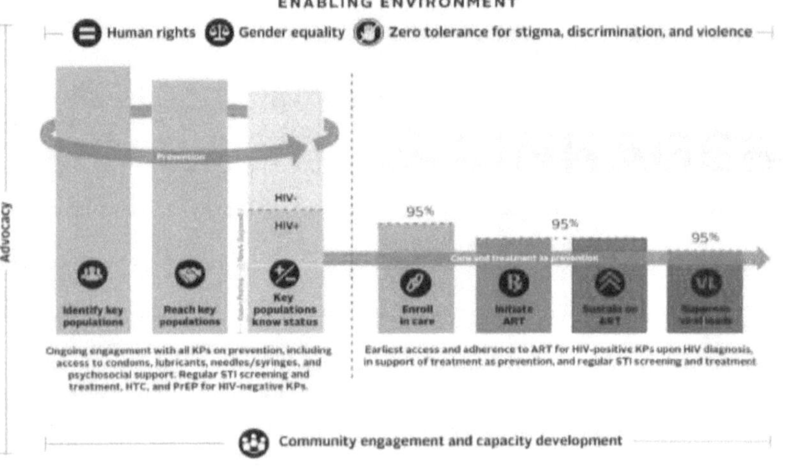

Figure 1. Cascade framework for HIV services along the continuum developed by Francis and Mills, 2005.

KPs key populations
STI sexually transmitted infections
HTC HIV testing and counseling
PrEP pre-exposure prophylaxis

6

Overall study design, steps and phases

The study methodology is divided in three steps: 1) initial program theory elicitation, 2) initial program theory testing through mixed method explanatory design and, 3) mechanisms identification and theory refinement (figure 2).

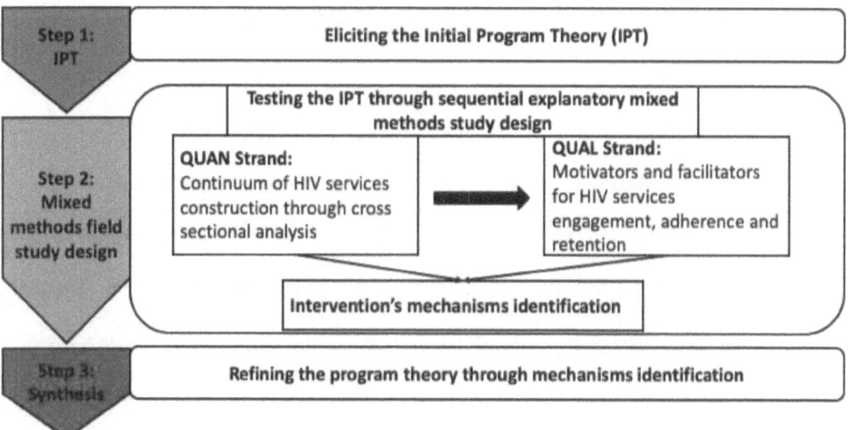

Figure 2. Study methodological process.

Step 1- Eliciting the IPT:

this evaluation started with the formulation of the IPT. We explored the development of the continuum by reviewing program framework and reports, discussing with program coordinators, healthcare providers and MSM and participant observations at the health facilities. Guided by realist evaluation principles, the findings were analyzed thematically. This IPT served as a hypothesis that was tested through a mixed methods design.

Step 2- Testing the IPT:

for this second step, we carried out a mixed methodology with a sequential explanatory design: a quantitative phase to build the continuum from a cross-sectional analysis, and a qualitative phase to explore the motivators and facilitators related to linkage along the continuum (20).

- Quantitative phase - Continuum construction and analysis:

A cross-sectional analysis from programmatic and technical reports data of activities implemented from January 2017 to December 2018 were used to construct the continuum. Then, to build the cohort, a retrospective review of MSM living with HIV electronic medical records (EMR) was used to collect data. As an exploratory part in nature no formal sample size calculations were conducted. Patients aged 18 years and above and enrolled between January 2017 and December 2018 were screened for eligibility to be included in the study. Patient files were excluded if they missed data on important variables including date for start of care, sexual orientation and age. We calculated the proportion of participants who proceeded through specific steps in the cascade from prevention to viral suppression. In January 2020, we calculated the outcomes for the cohort overall. This period ensured follow-up 12 months after enrolment. The events of interests were the number of MSM reached through prevention and testing services, who tested positive for HIV, were linked with HIV care, initiated ART, were retained in care (had at least two outpatient visits at least 90 days apart after ART initiation), had a viral load test at around 6 months after ART initiation, achieved viral suppression (less than 200 copies per mL), and were active and on treatment or lost to follow-up (180 days without any visit to clinic after starting ART) as described by the program specific objectives.

- Qualitative phase - Generating mechanisms and exploring pathways for engagement, adherence and retention:

We conducted 5 Key informants' interviews to explore how the program works. Then, 27 in-depth interviews (12 with MSM who were LTFU and 15 with MSM who were active and on ART) were also conducted to study the perceptions of MSM regarding the HIV care continuum, their experiences and the potential motivators and facilitators for engagement, adherence and retention. The key informants involved five doctors, program coordinators and MSM peer educators. In order to ensure maximum variation, we managed to elicit views from MSM patients enrolled in care and receiving ART and from MSM who were LTFU. Those LTFU were contacted using the telephone contact extracted from the EMR. All interviews were conducted in French Creole using an interview guide and were recorded and transcribed verbatim. Saturation was reached after conducting 27 in-depth interviews. Our inductive approach to data analysis was based on the thematic analysis in line with the study aim (21,22).

The methods were integrated through triangulation of quantitative analysis to assess the steps of the continuum and qualitative analysis to elicit mechanisms. While the retrospective cohort analysis provided an insight into the continuum of care and the outcomes of the MSM, the qualitative data analysis provided the evidence to strengthen every step in the cascade by identifying the mechanisms and pathways that can contribute to better outcomes

Step 3: Refining the program theory through mechanisms identification:
the aim of the third step was to identify mechanisms and pathways through an assessment of the continuum and a thematic content analysis. The IPT provided a basic framework on understanding how and why mechanisms generate the outcomes which are linkage to care, adherence and retention. Codes and themes were generated in regard to the context, mechanisms, pathways and intervention strategies in an iterative way.

Trustworthiness of the work

Prior to data collection and in order to understand the contextual factors relating to the HIV care continuum for MSM, meetings and observations were held with MSM patients, and healthcare workers. Credibility was established by selecting key informants' interviews and in-depth interviews to collect data while being familiar with the context. Dependability was established by describing the data analysis in detail and providing direct citations to reveal the basis from which the analysis was conducted. The citations used in this article were translated from French Creole into English with the help of a translator, to maintain accuracy and context as much as possible. Conformability and consistency of the analysis were established by holding meetings for the team to discuss preliminary findings, emerging codes and themes until consensus reached. To enhance the transferability of the findings, descriptions of contexts, selection of participants, data collection and analysis are provided in order to enable the readers the possibilities to determine whether the results of this study are transferable to another context (23,24).

Ethics statement

Authorization to conduct the study was obtained from the GHESKIO's human right committee and the Cornell University Weil Medical College's Research Ethics Board. At the level of the program, permission was obtained from the facility managers, and finally, consents from the participants and the key informants were obtained. Confidentiality was assured and data were anonymized.

Results

Step 1—Eliciting the IPT

The IPT described how the implemented interventions within Haitian specific healthcare and structural contexts have produced the expected outcomes. This is the result from reviews of the grey literature, program frameworks and project combined with assumptions by stakeholders about what inputs and processes are required to ensure linkages across the continuum regarding the context (8,25-27). As presented in the figure 3, developing the IPT allowed us to identify the inputs (governance, financing, personal, equipment, facilities and materials) behind the

10

Figure 4. The continuum of HIV services for MSM.

The demographic characteristics of the MSM who started ART are presented in Table 1. Most of them were in their 20s (n = 66, 52.8%) with secondary and superior education level n = 95, 76%). Nearly half of them were unemployed (n = 47, 37.6%) and with an income of less than $ 5.000 US / year (n = 62, 49.6%). Most participants reported having sexual partners (n = 121, 97.6%), however, only a few (n = 8, 6.7%) disclosed their HIV status to their sexual partners and used condom on a regular basis (n = 16, 13.3%). Most of the participants reported being married to women (n = 100, 80%).

He explained how it is easy for gays to be infected. At that particular moment, I realized that I've been at risk without knowing. This is why I am now a trainer, to help others understand that and participate in community meetings." [IDIMSM0004]

Pathway 3 - Acceptance and HIV status: although MSM reported a variety of feelings after their HIV diagnosis, they explained that being able to cope with their HIV status leads to self-acceptance, self-stigma mitigation and peer support seeking through disclosure.

"What could I do more? Nothing. I simply accept my result and I realized that I am also lucky to be able to receive treatment." [IDIMSM0011]

Mechanism 2: Sense of community support

Social relations among MSM represent a reliable source of better health outcomes. However, community stigma can impede the progress. Thus, increase social relation and empowerment lead to an established network essential to community education and awareness on issues linked to sexual orientation and HIV infection stigma and discrimination.

Pathway 4 - Addressing community stigma: according to the participants, community and family stigma have contributed to a large number of MSM refusing preventive care, missing their appointments in the clinic and discontinuing their treatment. Thus, community education and awareness on issues linked to sexual orientation and HIV infection play a major role in encouraging care-seeking behavior, adherence and retention.

"It is difficult to take the medications and come for appointments when everyone at your house and neighborhood don't accept the fact you are gay." [IDIMSM0014]

Pathway 5 - Strengthening of MSM organizations and community networks: the key informants and the MSM provided insights about the role of organizations and networks in promoting social activities to improve confidence and allow free exchange of ideas, coordination of participative projects towards achieving effective results in engaging MSM in prevention and care.

"We are having important help from the MSM networks. They help us reach other MSM and we are always invited to conduct training and counseling during their weekly meetings. If someone miss appointments, they call him or visit him…During the meetings they tell their own stories to motivate others" [KIICHW0002]

Pathway 6 - Societal acceptation and tolerance: MSM explained that highly stigmatized by both religious and social norms, their homosexual practices are driven underground. Besides, in some cases they face violence perpetuated at a community level. They advocated for better legal protections in order to promote tolerance which can decrease HIV vulnerability and increase access to sexual and HIV information, testing, prevention and care.

"If I don't feel safe in the community, I will not go to the activities." [IDIMSM0013]
"I was afraid to go in the meetings at first, but my friend picked me up, we go together, this is the reason why I stay." [IDIMSM0016]

Mechanism 3: Sense of comprehensive and tailored HIV services.

Sense of comprehensive and tailored HIV services represents a step towards trust and confidence in the health systems. It is a mechanism based on three different pathways: 1) stigma reduction training for healthcare providers, 2) engagement of peers as educators and navigators and, 3) adapted services delivery through drug dispensing points and mobile technology and 4) Financial assistance.

Pathway 7 - Sexual stigma reduction training for healthcare providers: some participants reported having experienced stigma when they interact with health workers, while participating in community initiatives and clinical activities. Therefore, they mentioned needs to properly deliver sexual stigma reduction training as a key to successful link to care.

"I think the nurses also need training to know how to talk to gays. I don't like the way they refer to me, or call me when I am waiting..." [IDIMSM0017]

Pathway 8 - Engagement of peers as educators, navigators, and treatment supporters: MSM and key informants recognized the importance of peer educators and navigators as important members of the team for essential prevention, and care promoting strategies. They specifically expressed their involvement in subtle and comprehensive discussions to change risky sexual behaviors and to increase adherence to care.

"I felt difficult to go there (hospital) at first. But, with the peer educator, I understood the reasons why it is important for me to take the medications, go to the appointments and protect my friends." [IDIMSM0012]

Pathway 9 - Adapted services delivery through drug dispensing points and mobile technology: in order to avoid long waiting time at the clinic and work time conflicts and absence due to the country political instability, the solutions that MSM proposed is to have adapted services where they are able to receive their drugs in other clinical settings, local pharmacies and community locations with respect to confidentiality.

"During the appointment, I mentioned the fact that I am working. Now, I receive a message on my phone to remind me of the appointment... I can come on Saturday...Since then, I have had no more problems with my director." [IDIMSM0008]

Pathway 10 - Financial assistance: as lack of employment represented a key factor to inability to afford indirect expenses such as transportation to the clinic for routine visits, MSM advocated for economic support such as transportation fees, decrease of visit frequency and implementation of mobile clinics.

"I missed some visits because I didn't have the money to go. But, since they started giving us the fees, it is so much easier for me to go.' [IDIMSM0006]

Step 3- Refining the program theory through mechanisms identification

The IPT provided a basic framework on understanding the limitations and barriers towards proper linkages and showed how and why mechanisms generate the outcomes. Therefore, we present an exploration of how, why, for whom, and in which circumstances particular mechanisms work. For each outcome, we tested the association with an identified mechanism and pathways taking into consideration the context. The CMO configuration was then refined during this process. Thus, figure 5 represent the refined program theory by using an interpretive approach to synthesize evidence to reveal how processes interact with context to trigger mechanisms in order to produce the outcomes.

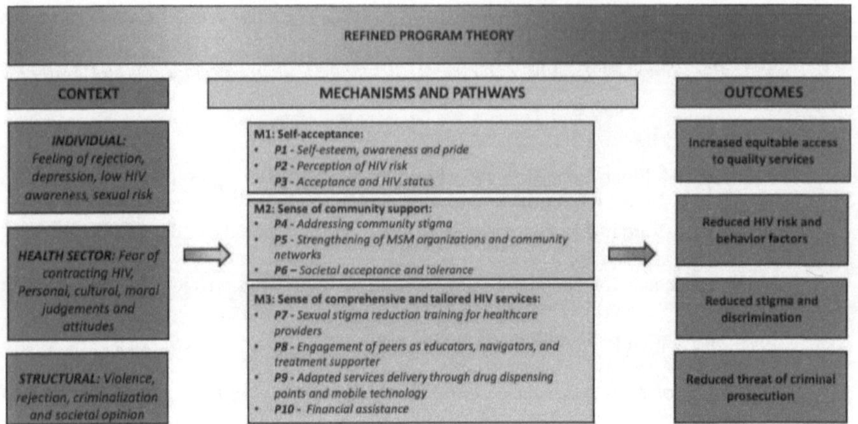

Figure 5. Refined program theory illustrating the mechanisms and pathways to engagement, adherence and retention throughout the continuum.

Discussion

Considering that programs are embedded theory, the use of realist method in this study allows us to conduct the evaluation while capturing the gaps between each step of the continuum, the contextual factors and a package of propositions for its improvement (28).

Since the beginning of the HIV epidemic, MSM have been one of the most at-risk groups (29). Due to many contextual factors, and particularly because they are subjected to self, perceived stigma and discrimination, proper engagement in health services is difficult (30). While many interventions have been tested for MSM, yet some struggle to accept and adjust to their HIV diagnosis, decided not to initiate ART and some are lost to follow-up (31). This study revealed the pattern for MSM in Haiti but also tried to identify relevant mechanisms to address those issues. We used a mixed-approach surrounded by a theory-based method to build the continuum and gain insights into motivators and facilitators to fill the gaps. Through quantitative assessment we build the continuum, identify the breaches, and qualitative exploration, we identified the pathways and mechanisms to achieve key milestones for overall improvement.

Our main findings proved that the current service delivery models are less than optimal in engaging and retaining MSM, resulting in lost to follow-up and failure to fully realize the health and prevention benefits of ART. However, we also explored valuable insights in identifying pathways lead to better engagement, adherence and retention through mechanisms identification. Our results demonstrate that the 95-95-95: the fast-track is far to be reached as MSM are lost from the prevention step. These findings were in accordance with other studies evaluating the continuum in many different contexts (32-34). However, some important considerations must be highlighted about these results: first, attracting MSM through community activities is difficult in a country where homosexuality is still largely disapproved; second, disclosure of sexual orientation during consultation is suboptimal; therefore, our data of MSM in care only represents patients who voluntarily disclosed their sexual orientation. In addition, viral suppression appears relatively acceptable among those who started ART even though many of them were already lost to follow-up.

We found that disclosure was rarely practiced by MSM. Only 6.7% reported disclosing their HIV-positive status to their partners while 98% don't use condom on a regular basis. Given the critical role of unprotected anal sex in HIV transmission, the low reported disclosure rate is concerning (35). Besides, 80% have already been married to a woman. Although some MSM may wish to engage in relationships with both men and women, heteronormative culture may lead MSM to marry women regardless of their preferences, concealing their same-sex behavior and placing their wives at risk of HIV. This gendered vulnerabilities that contribute to HIV-risk has also been reported in other settings (36).

The improvement of continuum of HIV services is a challenge everywhere. Interpersonal, intrapersonal, health system related and structural barriers are important impediments to goal achievement throughout the continuum (37). However, three sets of mechanisms embedded in ten pathways were identified according to the interviews. Self-acceptance through self-esteem, awareness and pride, perception of HIV risk and acceptance and HIV status is a key component on addressing the intrapersonal barriers. The MSM can be more confident by focusing on greater self-awareness of emotions, goals, behaviors, and associated barriers while fostering acceptance of parts of the self that cannot change. Sense of community support by addressing community stigma, strengthening of MSM organizations and community networks allow MSM to help their peers not only for stigma reduction but also for engagement and retention in care. Sense of comprehensive and tailored HIV services with sexual stigma reduction training for healthcare providers, engagement of peer support and adapted services delivery through drug dispensing points and mobile technology contribute to better comprehensive care. Enhance motivation and adaptation by societal acceptation, tolerance and financial assistance contribute to better continuum outcomes by enhancing motivation and adaptation throughout the dynamism of the specific context.

Refining the IPT by mechanism identification, it appears that interventions are more effective when multiple layers of strategies are implemented together to address complex health programs, such as the continuum of HIV services. Thus, our refined program theory provides sufficient evidence to claim that multi-level pathways are essential for continuum outcomes improvement. With the expanding recognition of the importance of the continuum of HIV services for MSM on decreasing HIV morbidity, mortality and transmission, engagement, adherence and retention play an important on achieving a generation free of HIV by 2030. It is crucial that relevant mechanisms and pathways are included in every step on developing interventions for MSM.

A key limitation of this realist evaluation is that we were very restricted by including MSM who voluntarily disclosed their sexual orientation from only one healthcare setting due to data quality and consistency. Additionally, it is likely that some of the views shared during the interviews are based on perceptions and not lived experiences. As a result, we may have missed some other contextual factors, mechanisms and pathways. However, the LINKAGE intervention represented a pilot effort in order to expand the strategy to the entire network of HIV care throughout the country. Thus, we propose that the mechanisms and pathway outlined in this paper should be seen as the essential, rather than the only one contributing to better continuum outcomes. Another limitation is that we were not able to fully capture the specific components of each step of the continuum. In order to be able to focus on the general aspects, we have purposively overlooked these stratifications at a global level. Despite these limitations, the use of a realist evaluation is increasingly relevant according to the conceptualization of the intervention. The mixed methodology used added value in trying to achieve a complete view from triangulation and saturation. Our findings provide valuable insight into the inconsistency of the continuum and the relevant pathways and mechanisms. Additionally, to the best of our knowledge this is the first time that realist evaluation has been used to assess HIV complex interventions in Haiti as this approach is more suitable for exploring complex interventions. The study findings show that engagement, adherence and retention to the continuum of HIV service for MSM are affected by a multi-layer of factors, thus highlighting the importance of taking a comprehensive approach to improve the program.

Abbreviations

IPT: Initial Program Theory; HIV: Human immunodeficiency virus; HIV/AIDS: Human immunodeficiency virus and Acquired immune deficiency syndrome; loss to follow-up: LTFU; MSM: Men who have Sex with Men; PLHIV: people living with HIV.

Authors' contributions

WD, AL, NM and YC conceived the original research idea and led the design of the study. WD, NM and AL collected the data. WD, AL and NM conducted the analysis. WD, AL, NM and YC provided insights in the final program theory. WD developed the first draft of the article. WD, AL, NM and YC oversaw the development of the article and contributed to the revisions. All authors reviewed and approved the final draft.

Acknowledgements

Authors would like to acknowledge Stéphano Saint-Preux and Schamir Prosper from the Haitian Study Group for Kaposi's Sarcoma and Opportunistic Infections (GHESKIO), Port-au-Prince, Haiti for their help in logistics, data collection and analysis during the study.

Competing interests

The authors declare that they have no competing interests.

8- Giordano, T., 2015. The HIV Treatment Cascade—A New Tool in HIV Prevention. *JAMA Internal Medicine*, 175(4), p.596.

9- Wong, N., Mao, J., Cheng, W., Tang, W., Cohen, M., Tucker, J. and Xu, H., 2017. HIV Linkage to Care and Retention in Care Rate Among MSM in Guangzhou, China. *AIDS and Behavior*, 22(3), pp.701-710.

10- Crowell, T., Keshinro, B., Baral, S., Schwartz, S., Stahlman, S., Nowak, R., Adebajo, S., Blattner, W., Charurat, M. and Ake, J., 2017. Stigma, access to healthcare, and HIV risks among men who sell sex to men in Nigeria. *Journal of the International AIDS Society*, 20(1), p.21489.

11- Rouzier, V., Farmer, P., Pape, J., Jerome, J., Van Onacker, J., Morose, W., Joseph, P., Leandre, F., Severe, P., Barry, D., Deschamps, M. and Koenig, S., 2014. Factors impacting the provision of antiretroviral therapy to people living with HIV: the view from Haiti. *Antiviral Therapy*, 19(Suppl 3), pp.91-104.

12- Daniels, J., 2019. Haiti's complex history with HIV, and recent successes. *The Lancet HIV*, 6(3), pp.e151-e152.

13- Zalla, L., Herce, M., Edwards, J., Michel, J. and Weir, S., 2019. The burden of HIV among female sex workers, men who have sex with men and transgender women in Haiti: results from the 2016 Priorities for Local AIDS Control Efforts (PLACE) study. *Journal of the International AIDS Society*, 22(7).

14- Nelson, K., Thiede, H., Jenkins, R., Carey, J., Hutcheson, R. and Golden, M., 2014. Personal and Contextual Factors Related to Delayed HIV Diagnosis Among Men Who Have Sex With Men. *AIDS Education and Prevention*, 26(2), pp.122-133.

15- Dalkin, S., Greenhalgh, J., Jones, D., Cunningham, B. and Lhussier, M., 2015. What's in a mechanism? Development of a key concept in realist evaluation. *Implementation Science*, 10(1).

16- Pawson, R., 2004. Simple Principies for the Evaluation of Complex Programmes. *CIDADES, Comunidades e Territórios*, (8).

17- Pawson, R., 2002. Evidence-based Policy: The Promise of `Realist Synthesis'. *Evaluation*, 8(3), pp.340-358.

18- Triana, R., 2008. Evidence-Based Policy: A Realist Perspective, by Ray Pawson. *Journal of Policy Practice*, 7(4), pp.321-323.

19- Pawson, R., 2014. A realist approach to qualitative research Joseph A Maxwell. *Qualitative Social Work*, 13(4), pp.585-586.

20- Ozawa, S. and Pongpirul, K., 2013. 10 best resources on … mixed methods research in health systems. *Health Policy and Planning*, 29(3), pp.323-327.

21- Creswell, J., & Plano Clark, V. (2007). Designing and Conducting Mixed Methods Research. Thousand Oaks, CA: Sage. *Organizational Research Methods*, 12(4), pp.801-804.

22- McKim, C., 2016. The Value of Mixed Methods Research. *Journal of Mixed Methods Research*, 11(2), pp.202-222.

23- Korstjens, I. and Moser, A., 2017. Series: Practical guidance to qualitative research. Part 4: Trustworthiness and publishing. *European Journal of General Practice*, 24(1), pp.120-124.

24- Cypress, B., 2017. Rigor or Reliability and Validity in Qualitative Research. *Dimensions of Critical Care Nursing*, 36(4), pp.253-263.

25- Needle, R., Fu, J., Beyrer, C., Loo, V., Abdul-Quader, A., McIntyre, J., Li, Z., Mbwambo, J., Muthui, M. and Pick, B., 2012. PEPFAR's Evolving HIV Prevention Approaches for Key Populations—People Who Inject Drugs, Men Who Have Sex With Men, and Sex Workers. *JAIDS Journal of Acquired Immune Deficiency Syndromes*, 60(Supplement 3), pp.S145-S151.

PART 4. DISCUSSIONS

Aims of the book

The purpose of this book was: to analyze the continuum of HIV services for MSM in order to ascertain why, how and under which circumstances MSM are engaged, linked and retained along the care continuum; to identify loss to follow-up throughout the continuum by comparing the initial objectives of the program and achievements; to identify the socio-demographic and clinical profiles of the MSM who have left the continuum while exploring the context; to assess the barriers and facilitators to engagement, adherence and retention along the continuum while identifying the underlying mechanisms; to evaluate the impact of perceived, enacted and experienced stigma by MSM in healthcare structures; and, to generate essential information for participatory revision of socially accountable procedures in order to improve the outcomes.

The objectives were driven by those following questions: how to ensure proper engagement, adherence and retention along the continuum of HIV services for MSM, what are the proportions of LTFU in each step of the continuum, what are the sociodemographic and clinical profiles of the MSM retained and lost, what are the underlying mechanisms of barriers and facilitators to engagement, adherence and retention along the continuum, and how perceived, enacted and experienced stigma affect the continuum?

Synthesis of the findings

A summary of the findings indicates that MSM experienced stigma in multiple and overlapping layers. In general terms, people living with HIV know that their status is an extremely socially devalued aspect of the self, and this knowledge is experienced through at least three important stigma forms: enacted stigma, anticipated stigma, and internalized stigma. Enacted stigma refers to the degree to which people believe they have actually experienced prejudice and discrimination from others in their community. Anticipated stigma refers to the degree to which people expect that they will experience prejudice and discrimination from others in the future. Internalized stigma refers to the degree to which people endorse the negative beliefs and feelings associated with HIV/AIDS about themselves (1).

In our studies, MSM described stigmatizing experiences stemming from religious sources, communities, family and friends, and from the medical establishment. From the social construction of heteronormativity in the society, several social and cultural factors, gender norms lie behind the stigma associated with sexual orientation and HIV (2). Moreover, medical students and healthcare givers still carry discriminatory attitudes towards them despite tailored interventions (3).

Our analysis showed that current service delivery models are less than optimal in linking and retaining MSM, resulting in loss to follow-up in the continuum of care and failure to fully realize the health and prevention benefits (4,5). However, multi-level, contextual-based and socially accountable interventions can produce stigma mitigation through personal, health systems' and contextual mechanisms for better engagement, adherence and retention throughout the continuum.

Suitability of the realist approach

In this study, the use of realist review and evaluation allowed us to evaluate stigma on different angles and to capture the continuum's gaps as well as the relevance of multilevel factors in shaping the MSM engagement, adherence and retention (6–8). Realist methodology has been considered to be well suited for evaluating complex interventions, as it allows for analyzing interactions between different layers of context, outcomes and the underlying mechanisms (9). The overall methodology applied allowed us to describe the contexts, elicit the mechanisms and enable the outcomes through a thoughtful succession of steps from scoping and systematic literature reviews, qualitative and mixed methods explanatory researches. This approach also showed the importance of context which is often not fully considered while implementing and evaluating public health interventions (10). However, the results are from a combination of dynamic equation between the specific context, health systems and policies in Haiti. Needless to say that findings from this book may not be fully appropriate to other contexts.

Discussions of the main results while considering other studies:

Epidemiology of HIV in MSM populations

The epidemiology of HIV in MSM populations showed the direct links with many implications for prevention, treatment, retention and follow-up. From the published data, HIV prevalence in MSM population is 18% compared to 2% among the general population (5). Even with great variations, the high prevalence and rate of new infections among MSM require more vigorous, scientifically informed and tailored responses. As MSM are 27 times more at risk for HIV and 23% of new infections were among them in 2019, the development and implementation of strategies to address the high biological risks associated with anal sex are urgently needed (10-12).

Although, the epidemiology is well known, available data to calculate prevalence and incidence in MSM remain incomplete and various settings including Haiti (13). Four decades after discovering HIV, more than 50 countries have no available reports on MSM or when published, such reports are hampered by the lack of population-based measures of the prevalence of same-sex behaviors in men, the size of the populations at risk, and the great diversity of these populations in differing social, cultural, and political contexts. Besides, social response biases against reporting some behaviors, including receptive anal sex, are likely to affect risk factor assessment (14). Size estimation approaches must be revised. One of the major issues in controlling the epidemics among MSM is he disparity in number of HIV cases among them compared to population size that has been difficult to quantify and poorly studied (12, 13). Even in Haiti, while the national statistics data currently allow the health sector to calculate disease rates by key variables including sex at birth and age, there are no census data for the number of MSM in Haiti. Estimation of a population size for MSM is crucial in allowing the calculation of disease rates among them as well as the possibility to quantify the disparate impact of various diseases among MSM and to better guide program interventions. Encouragingly, these limitations have led to a range of innovations in epidemiology and are proving of use to the description of other hidden, stigmatized, or otherwise hard-to-reach populations (15).

Stigma: assessment and impact

Described from our studies and reported by other research, opinions about sexuality and homosexuality comprise part of the structural factors that influence a country's response to its HIV epidemic. Thus, evidence from our work indicates that stigma meets all of the criteria to be considered as a fundamental barrier to the steps across the continuum of HIV services (4,5). Reducing HIV prevalence among MSM remains one of the most critical challenges in effectively controlling the HIV epidemic. Worldwide, critical challenges and gaps remain which are impeding the identification of effective stigma-reduction strategies that can be implemented on a larger scale (11,12).

While clinical and community level interventions remained the most common in those countries including Haiti, some community-level efforts have been tested in small groups and a few interventions at the organizational-level have been planned, realized and studied (13,14). HIV prevention programs aimed at sexual minority groups are mindful of potentially complex relationships between social stigmas such as homophobia and sexual risk-taking behaviour. However, it is unlikely that this will set the feasibility with the current methods of prevention and treatment unless significant progress is made in reducing the strong stigma associated with homosexuality, removing the structural barriers to them accessing social services, addressing their social vulnerability, and empowering them to practice safe sex (15). A clear response to improve the legal/human rights environment affecting sexual diversity is urgently needed, not only on grounds of progress of the international agenda on human rights, but also based on a public health and development perspective. Multisectoral efforts should be made to show the social harm of homophobic laws and practices, and to generate initiatives leading to positive changes (16,17).

While Haiti has relatively tolerant laws relating to homosexuality, the recent adoption of a law against same-sex marriages by the Haitian Senate appears to reflect the high level of homophobia in the country and our works showed that it is impeding the future Haitian HIV response (18–20). Through various activities, the Government of Haiti is strongly committed to reducing HIV among MSM. The Ministère de la Santé Publique et de la Population, alongside with other organizations, has set HIV programs for MSM and other Key Populations through the national strategic plan. Training on stigma and discrimination among HCW was also conducted and has targeted public health workers and health staff of implementing partners. Despite those actions, the response remained weak as many barriers persist including stigma and discrimination (3,21,22). Those findings are in line with other studies conducted in countries around the world and with similar and different contexts (17,23,24).

In our assessment of the impact of stigma and discrimination on the continuum, we found that stigma measurement tools continue to be an important issue. The majority of studies examining MSM stigma have included a focus on sexual orientation constructs and the use of anti-gay/anti-homosexuality attitude scales. While many researchers highlighted the importance of scales, it is crucial to adapt the tools when measuring stigma affecting MSM who do not self-identify as gay or homosexual, particularly in Haiti and other countries with different local terms and identities that do not fit easily into the MSM paradigm. The lack of standardized measurement tools for stigma and discrimination greatly limits our way to design and judge which strategies work the best for addressing the various stigma domains or targeting different socio-ecological levels (26–28). The development of validated measures assessing each domain of the stigmatization process must be a priority in order to shift with programmatic efforts and/or structural interventions (7). However, this work found a few validated scales created for measuring MSM-associated stigma and some others adapted for the studies. The availability of tested stigma-reduction tools and approaches needs to be improved (1).

Stigma in healthcare settings

A further reflection needs to be done on the weakness between homosexuality and the attention given by healthcare professional and healthcare students. MSM experience difficulties engaging in care, disclosing their behaviors and adhering due to the embarrassing situations when expressing their homosexuality/bisexuality (3,29,30). The qualitative study conducted to explore their attitudes regarding MSM revealed three main findings: a) participants expressed their willingness to provide MSM with comprehensive healthcare; b) medical education curriculum does not consider MSM-specific sexual health and emerging layered stigma attitudes while providing comprehensive services through discussion about same-sex relationship; and c) suggestions of a more inclusive medical education and non-judgmental, caring attitudes of professors and clinical instructors. While students feel the obligation to provide care to MSM like any other patient, some of them would not be comfortable. They clearly indicated that they did not have the requisite skills necessary to handle MSM health specificities; most of them felt that they not only needed to be clinically trained, effective communication training sessions needed to be delivered to their professors (3).

Evidence of the link between health training institutions and communities has been around for a long time; however, it is only in recent decades that social accountability of health education has become more formalized (31,32). The "social contract" defines the duties of the training institutions with regard to all aspects of the societies in which they are established and where they draw their resources. It follows that training of health care providers will lead to skill improvement for quality of healthcare; however, efforts to shift attitudes have to consider the cultural components of the society (33).

Thus, solutions and strategies that gradually stimulate the adaptation of health professions to the realities of every community, including MSM, are necessary to strengthen professional ethics for the respect of rights, duties and freedom without stigma. Important revisions of curricula to introduce this topic in health sciences undergraduate's curricula; conducting training with already working professionals; monitoring the capacity-building interventions are needed. Homophobia represents a major barrier to accessing HIV services among MSM. They also have limited access to specialised programmes, even in comparison with people who inject drugs and sex workers. Moreover, programmes focused on clinical interventions need to also consider human right issues (34,35).

Elicited mechanisms from the realist review and evaluation

In order to elicit the mechanisms for stigma mitigation and continuum outcomes improvement, we conducted a realist review and realist evaluation of the continuum of HIV services (1).

The findings from the review helped us highlight the mechanisms through which stigma can be mitigated. Self-acceptance, leadership and motivational activation for behaviour change is a key component to intrapersonal strategies. MSM felt more confident and this mechanism is built by sharing a focus on greater self-awareness of emotions, goals, behaviours and associated barriers while fostering acceptance of parts of the self that cannot change. Socialization, knowledge sharing and social empowerment allow MSM to help their peers not only for stigma reduction but also for engagement and retention to care. Training sessions for caregivers allow them to better understand the specificities of MSM and allow them to have appropriate knowledge. Community introspection, self-reflection and humanistic activation allow structural changes through community engagement (1).

The realist evaluation showed three sets of mechanisms embedded in ten pathways. Self-acceptance through self-esteem, awareness and pride, perception of HIV risk and acceptance and HIV status is a key component in addressing the intrapersonal barriers. The MSM can be more confident by focusing on greater self-awareness of emotions, goals, behaviours, and associated barriers while fostering acceptance of parts of the self that cannot change. Sense of community support by addressing community stigma, societal acceptance and tolerance, strengthening of MSM organizations and community networks allow MSM to help their peers not only for stigma reduction but also for engagement and retention in care. Sense of comprehensive and tailored HIV services with sexual stigma reduction training for healthcare providers, engagement of peer support, financial assistance, and adapted services delivery through drug dispensing points and mobile technology contribute to better comprehensive care.

Several intervention strategies, such as the training for HCPs and religious leaders, show how specific training sessions lead to changes in stigmatizing attitudes and behaviours against MSM. These strategies, however, do not sufficiently consider intrapersonal mechanisms of stigma generation. It appears that stigma interventions are more effective when multiple strategies are implemented together to address complex health programs, such as the HIV prevention and care continuum. Our model provides sufficient evidence to claim that multi-level intervention strategies are essential for stigma mitigation (1,5).

Political will and resources to support and scale up stigma reduction activities throughout health care settings (1-3). Based on such understanding, public messaging, communications and educational campaigns can be reshaped and targeted more effectively for the elimination of stigma and discrimination, resulting in a more efficient, equitable and acceptable HIV response (10). Interventions including "safe" spaces for MSM to be educated and to obtain information are crucial (11).

Our work showed a strong evidence that HIV interventions for MSM need to be tailored according to the dynamism of the contexts with respect to cultural and structural values. Few MSM can find respectful and high-quality HIV services to stay healthy and safe by engaging, adhering and retaining in those services. This book provides a unique opportunity to build comprehensive interventions strategies from theory-based mechanisms. Yet, many challenges still persist including limited systems capacity, stigma and discrimination, violence, discriminatory attitudes and other social norms that reduce access to resources and result in low social status, exclusion of MSM from meaningful input, and lack of government support to scale up and sustain MSM services currently funded by donors. With respect to the existed intervention strategies, those mechanisms and pathway contribute to offer MSM living with and at risk for HIV:

- Self-motivation to access better quality and more integrated HIV services.
- Confidentiality protection.
- Peer support on accessing the steps of the continuum.
- Understanding needs in a non-stigmatizing way.
- Community tolerance.

- Meaningful opportunities for community engagement.

Strategic framework for stigma mitigation

Converted into strategies, the mechanisms are listed based on a comprehensive classification: intrapersonal, interpersonal, health systems-based and structural.

Intrapersonal strategies
Education for MSM
As part of the intrapersonal strategies, education for MSM represented a key strategy for stigma reduction. Education provides opportunities both to learn about sexuality and to express feelings through social activities. To illustrate, the education method adopted a family structure that also serves as a refuge for MSM while providing social support and guidance. With a decline in stigma, this strategy may lead to empowerment on using natural leadership skills to influence friends and acquaintances to protect themselves from HIV.

Mobile and online health interventions
Online strategies to reduce stigma have two components: addressing feelings of shame and increasing interactive discussion. Strategies that act against shame associated with sexual stigma by enabling MSM to more consciously acknowledge their desires and to recognize that their desires are normal. With sexual shame reduction unprotected anal intercourses may also be indirectly decreased. Shame reduction is an important intervention component resulting in HIV prevention and care enrolment.

Individual-motivational interviewing counselling (IMIC)
Associated with sexual risk reduction and improvement in HIV stigma, IMIC is a collaborative, client-centred counselling style designed to increase motivational readiness to behaviour change by exploring ambivalence about change, eliciting discrepancies between current behaviours and personal goals, and building self-efficacy.

Self-esteem, awareness and pride
Self-esteem, awareness and pride are prominent determinants for mental health and well-being. Thus, those factors are precursors that play a significant role on steps to accept sexual

orientation. Psychosocial constructs are mandatory to improve willingness for overall health and therefore for HIV prevention and care engagement.

Perception of HIV risk

Even with fear of unintended disclosure and anticipated stigma, it is now recognized that basic knowledge of a higher potential and vulnerability for contracting HIV among MSM represents a key factor for taking part in HIV prevention and testing activities.

Acceptance and HIV status

Although HIV diagnosis may lead to a variety of feelings, being able to cope with HIV status leads to self-acceptance, self-stigma mitigation and peer support seeking through disclosure.

Interpersonal strategies

Support group meeting

With indoor and outdoor activities, this strategy promotes knowledge sharing, socializing between MSM and helps them to better prepare for and mitigate the effects of stigma and prejudice. Another form of support group meeting is to address issues of disclosure of sexual orientation, family rejection, and issues relating to oppression for MSM. Discussions allow for cultural nuances to shine through and after participation, safer sex behaviours, comfort disclosing sexual orientation and support from friends are reinforced. The implication is that HIV prevention needs to incorporate cultural, social, and structural factors.

Strengthening of MSM organizations and community networks

Organizations and networks play a crucial role in promoting social activities to improve confidence and allow free exchange of ideas, coordination of participative projects towards achieving effective results in engaging MSM in prevention and care.

Health Systems Strategies

Peer support, peer navigator

To operationalize a referral system, between peers, designed to provide users anonymous and real-time feedback and recommendations for where friendly, non-stigmatizing health services may be accessed.

Training for Healthcare providers

Aim at addressing enacted stigma and alleviating barriers to care for MSM on the part of the health care providers. It improves the clinical and social competency of the providers in addressing the needs of MSM. Topics include sex, sexuality, and sexual health; mental health promotion; overcoming barriers; creating a friendlier environment; health implications of sexual practices; assessing health status; evidence-based interventions; clinical care for HIV and other sexually transmitted infections; gender-based violence; and reproductive health.

Adapted services delivery through drug dispensing points and mobile technology

In order to avoid long waiting times at the clinic and work time conflicts and absence due to the country's political instability, adapted services where MSM are able to receive their drugs in other clinical settings, local pharmacies and community locations with respect to confidentiality are recommended.

Teaching social accountability through structural, sexual and cultural contexts

Evidence of the link between health training institutions and communities has been around for a long time; however, it is only in recent decades that social accountability of health education has become more formalized. The "social contract" defines the duties of the training institutions with regard to all aspects of the societies in which they are established and where they draw their resources. Thus, solutions and strategies that gradually stimulate the adaptation of health professions to the realities of every community, including MSM, are necessary to strengthen professional ethics for the respect of rights, duties and freedom without stigma.

Structural Strategies

Community-based activities

With several modules, community-based activities aim to cover topics like HIV prevention and transmission; human rights; stigma and discrimination; reproductive health; and living with HIV. Topics include HIV transmission and prevention, and risk reduction techniques; definitions of human rights and rights issues in the MSM community; and methods for identifying and responding to stigma and discrimination, stress management, and self-esteem. Additional topics may also include sexual health, nutrition specific information for PLHIV, disease progression, well-being, and life balance.

Training workshops for religious and community leaders

Workshop to address the following topics: MSM and HIV; stigma; identity, coming out and disclosure; anal sex and common sexual practices; HIV and sexually transmitted infections; mental health, anxiety, depression and substance abuse; HIV prevention measures; and risk reduction counselling. Approaches for reducing stigma can generate introspection and self-reflection in order to gradually apply more humanistic and caring discourse.

Addressing community stigma

Community education and awareness on issues linked to sexual orientation and HIV infection play a major role in encouraging care-seeking behaviour, adherence and retention.

Financial assistance

As lack of employment represents a key factor to inability to afford indirect expenses such as transportation to the clinic for routine visits, economic support such as transportation fees, decrease of visit frequency and implementation of mobile clinics are suitable.

Stigma and discrimination, major challenges still remain as moderate progress has been made in prevention and treatment; significant gaps remain to reach the 90-90-90 and to jump into the 95-95-95 targets set by the UNAIDS for 2030 (36); political instability and social unrest hamper supply chain and continuity. To enable improvement across the continuum, comprehensive, ostentatious, tailored and sustainable strategies need to be deployed in order to:

- Identify and quantify MSM populations while assessing risk and service access.
- Determine weakness and reveal access barriers across the continuum
- Scale up pathways and ensure adaptation through structural complexity.
- Address health services related barriers and transform engage MSM networks.
- Ensure comprehensive interventions are sustainable and adaptable over the course of time.
- Enlist support from leadership at the highest levels.
- Ensure legal protections for MSM.
- Integrate pre-exposure prophylaxis (PrEP) into existing healthcare systems and providers, such as primary care providers.

- Create a careful and comprehensive public messaging campaign to provide accurate and context-adapted community education.
- Train healthcare providers at all levels.
- Make screening tests and medications available at all levels to assure follow-up.
- Identify funding for integrated program roll-out, evaluation and research.

Limitations and strengths

In terms of limitations regarding this book, to describe stigma, life sciences and biomedical literature were reviewed but other relevant sources, particularly relating to socio-anthropological, policy, and legal analyses, may not have been captured. So, we may have missed some aspects of the socio-cultural contexts and mechanisms as well.

Another limitation is the subjective aspect of qualitative form of analysis and data interpretation through the process even if discussions to reach consensus were central among the team. Because of that, we were not specific in defining which particular interventions or the components of the intervention were more effective when generating the mechanisms. This limitation is also present in our realist evaluation during which we were restricted by including MSM who voluntarily disclosed their sexual orientation from only one healthcare setting due to data quality and consistency. Nevertheless, it is important that efforts to reach MSM do not overlook more hidden sub-categories who may only socialize and engage in a hidden way.

Additionally, it is likely that some of the views shared during the interviews are based on perceptions and not lived experiences. In the qualitative study that explored attitudes of medical students towards MSM living with HIV, the results represent the views from one medical school in Haiti; this may limit generalizability of the study findings. However, we tried to improve external validity by selecting participants from different backgrounds and cultures. Our study did not evaluate a respondent's level of practice during medical education to determine whether attitudes changed with increased amount of experience. However, the description of acceptability to provide HIV-related health services among students as elicited in this study could be valid in another setting with similar context.

On a general note, findings show that linkage, adherence and retention to the continuum of HIV service for MSM are affected by a multi-layer of factors, thus highlighting the importance of taking comprehensive approaches to improve the program.

Conclusion

As realist methodology seeks not to judge but to explain, and is driven by the question 'What works for whom in what circumstances and in what respects' we found that the elicited mechanisms and pathways in the refined program theories act complementarity and can be adapted in terms of different socio-structural and cultural contexts in which MSM exposed to and living with HIV are living. Thus, this work recommends improvement and strengthening of comprehensive health and social systems for planning, monitoring, evaluating and assuring the quality of HIV and global health services for MSM.

The findings from this book will establish their utility as they are translated into action for public health purposes such as program and policies design and evaluation. Resources must be directed to the populations at highest risk and to strategies that are cost-effective. During this doctoral pathway, we dealt with uncertainties and crisis due to political and civil unrest in Haiti and the global pandemic of covid-19. In effort to address these issues we had to make changes to the initial study protocol to stay on track while embracing the complexity of the work through continuous adaptation. The path through this PhD has been long and filled with concurrences and controversies; Parts of those concurrences and controversies may largely be over or not in public and global health communities, but the work of questioning, exploring, assessing, disseminating, implementing and evaluating has just begun; We still have a long way to go to combat stigma, discrimination, ostracism, injustice in order to restore tolerance and respect; Every effort matter in order to apply intersectional lens to give visibility to marginalized populations; Above all, anything that seems inalterable can change, nothing can be taken for granted and everything is possible.

References

1. Dunbar, W. *et al.* A realist systematic review of stigma reduction interventions for HIV prevention and care continuum outcomes among men who have sex with men. *International Journal of STD & AIDS* **31,** 712–723 (2020).

2. Dunbar, W., Pape, J. W. & Coppieters, Y. HIV among men who have sex with men in the Caribbean: reaching the left behind. *Revista Panamericana de Salud Pública* **45,** 1 (2021).

3. Dunbar, W., Alcide, C., Raccurt, C., Pape, J. W. & Coppieters, Y. Attitudes of medical students towards men who have sex with men living with HIV: implications for social

accountability. *International Journal of Medical Education* **11,** 233–239 (2020).

4. Dunbar W, Sohler N, Coppieters Y. Loss to follow up among men who have sex with men and heterosexual men living with HIV in Haiti. *European Journal of Public Health* **30,** (2020).

5. Dunbar, W., Sohler, N. & Coppieters, Y. Outcomes along the HIV continuum of care for Men who have Sex with Men in Haiti. *European Journal of Public Health* **30,** (2020).

6. Pawson, R. & Sridharan, S. Theory-driven evaluation of public health programmes. *Evidence-based Public Health* 43–62 (2009). doi:10.1093/acprof:oso/9780199563623.003.04

7   Pawson, R. & Tilley, N. Realistic Evaluation Bloodlines. *American Journal of Evaluation* **22,** 317–324 (2001).

8   Pawson, R., Greenhalgh, T., Harvey, G. & Walshe, K. Realist review - a new method of systematic review designed for complex policy interventions. *Journal of Health Services Research & Policy* **10,** 21–34 (2005).

9. Triana, R. Evidence-Based Policy: A Realist Perspective, by Ray Pawson. *Journal of Policy Practice* **7,** 321–323 (2008).

10. Korstjens, I. & Moser, A. Series: Practical guidance to qualitative research. Part 2: Context, research questions and designs. *European Journal of General Practice* **23,** 274–279 (2017).

11. Rodríguez-Madera, S. & Varas-Díaz, N. Puerto Rican Heterosexual Serodiscordant Couples. *HIV Prevention with Latinos* 227–244 (2012). doi:10.1093/acprof:oso/9780199764303.003.0013

12. Rogers, S. J. *et al.* Layered stigma among health-care and social service providers toward key affected populations in Jamaica and The Bahamas. *AIDS Care* **26,** 538–546 (2013).

13. Bui, T. C. *et al.* Sexual Motivation, Sexual Transactions and Sexual Risk Behaviors in Men who have Sex with Men in Dar es Salaam, Tanzania. *AIDS and Behavior* **18,** 2432–2441 (2014).

14. Logie, C. H. *et al.* Social–ecological factors associated with HIV infection among men who have sex with men in Jamaica. *International Journal of STD & AIDS* **29,** 80–88 (2017).

15. Mac-Seing, M. *et al.* Make visible the invisible: innovative strategies for the future of global health. *BMJ Global Health* **4,** (2019).

16. Alvarez-Jimenez, M. *et al.* On the HORYZON: Moderated online social therapy for

long-term recovery in first episode psychosis. *Schizophrenia Research* **143**, 143–149 (2013).

17.   Hladik, W. *et al.* Men Who Have Sex with Men in Kampala, Uganda: Results from a Bio-Behavioral Respondent Driven Sampling Survey. *AIDS and Behavior* **21**, 1478–1490 (2016).

18.   Figueroa, J. P. The Critical Role of Locally Conducted Research in Guiding the Response to the HIV Epidemic in Jamaica. *West Indian Medical Journal* **61**, 387–395 (2012).

19.   Deschamps, M.-M., Fitzgerald, D. W., Pape, J. W. & Johnson, W. D. HIV infection in Haiti: natural history and disease progression. *AIDS* **14**, 2515–2521 (2000).

20.   Dube F. Key Populations in Haiti. *United Nations Population Fund* Available at: https://www.unfpa.org/publications. (Accessed: 16th March 2021)

21.   Zalla, L. C., Herce, M. E., Edwards, J. K., Michel, J. & Weir, S. S. The burden of HIV among female sex workers, men who have sex with men and transgender women in Haiti: results from the 2016 Priorities for Local AIDS Control Efforts (PLACE) study. *Journal of the International AIDS Society* **22**, (2019).

22.   HIV prevalence among FSWs and MSM in Haiti. Available at: https://www.paho.org/hq/index.php?option=com_docman&view=download&category _slug=vigilancia-poblaciones-clave-4737&alias=19315-haiti-vigilancia-epidemiologica-vih-315&Itemid=270&lang=en. (Accessed: 13th March 2021)

23.   Zahn, R. *et al.* Human Rights Violations among Men Who Have Sex with Men in Southern Africa: Comparisons between Legal Contexts. *PLOS ONE* **11**, (2016).

24.   Quinn, K. & Dickson-Gomez, J. Homonegativity, Religiosity, and the Intersecting Identities of Young Black Men Who Have Sex with Men. *AIDS and Behavior* **20**, 51–64 (2015).

25.   Muzyamba, C., Broaddus, E. & Campbell, C. "You cannot eat rights": a qualitative study of views by Zambian HIV-vulnerable women, youth and MSM on human rights as public health tools. *BMC International Health and Human Rights* **15**, (2015).

26.   Christensen, J. L. *et al.* Reducing shame in a game that predicts HIV risk reduction for young adult men who have sex with men: a randomized trial delivered nationally over the web. *Journal of the International AIDS Society* **16**, 18716 (2013).

27.   van der Elst, E. M. *et al.* The green shoots of a novel training programme: progress and identified key actions to providing services to MSM at Kenyan health facilities. *Journal of the International AIDS Society* **18**, 20226 (2015).

28. Stangl, A. L., Lloyd, J. K., Brady, L. M., Holland, C. E. & Baral, S. A systematic review of interventions to reduce HIV-related stigma and discrimination from 2002 to 2013: how far have we come? *Journal of the International AIDS Society* **16,** 18734 (2013).

29. Earnshaw, V. A. & Chaudoir, S. R. From Conceptualizing to Measuring HIV Stigma: A Review of HIV Stigma Mechanism Measures. *AIDS and Behavior* **13,** (2009).

30. Morris, M. *et al.* Training to reduce LGBTQ-related bias among medical, nursing, and dental students and providers: a systematic review. *BMC Medical Education* **19,** (2019).

31. Tudrej, B. V. La responsabilité sociale des facultés de médecine, un moyen de réconcilier les étudiants avec leur engagement médical. *Pédagogie Médicale* **14,** 73–74 (2013).

32. Boelen, C. Coordinating medical education and health care systems: the power of the social accountability approach. *Medical Education* **52,** 96–102 (2017).

33. Boelen, C. & Woollard, B. Social accountability and accreditation: a new frontier for educational institutions. *Medical Education* **43,** 887–894 (2009).

34. Beyrer, C. *et al.* A call to action for comprehensive HIV services for men who have sex with men. *The Lancet* **380,** 424–438 (2012).

35. Logie, C. H. *et al.* Social–ecological factors associated with HIV infection among men who have sex with men in Jamaica. *International Journal of STD & AIDS* **29,** 80–88 (2017).

36. 2016 United Nations Political Declaration on Ending AIDS sets world on the Fast-Track to end the epidemic by 2030. *UNAIDS Viet Nam 2016 United Nations Political Declaration on Ending AIDS sets world on the FastTrack to end the epidemic by 2030 Comments* Available at: https://unaids.org.vn/2016-united-nations-political-declaration-ending-aids-sets-world-fast-track-end-epidemic-2030/.